Clinical Manual for Diagnosis and Treatment of Psychotic Depression

Clinical Manual for Diagnosis and Treatment of Psychotic Depression

Anthony J. Rothschild, M.D.
Irving S. and Betty Brudnick Endowed Chair and
Professor of Psychiatry, Department of Psychiatry
University of Massachusetts Medical School
UMass Memorial Health Care
Worcester, Massachusetts

American Psychiatric Publishing, Inc.

Washington, DC
London, England

Note: The author has worked to ensure that all information in this book is accurate at the time of publication and consistent with general psychiatric and medical standards, and that information concerning drug dosages, schedules, and routes of administration is accurate at the time of publication and consistent with standards set by the U.S. Food and Drug Administration and the general medical community. As medical research and practice continue to advance, however, therapeutic standards may change. Moreover, specific situations may require a specific therapeutic response not included in this book. For these reasons and because human and mechanical errors sometimes occur, we recommend that readers follow the advice of physicians directly involved in their care or the care of a member of their family.

Books published by American Psychiatric Publishing, Inc., represent the views and opinions of the individual authors and do not necessarily represent the policies and opinions of APPI or the American Psychiatric Association.

Manufactured in the United States of America on acid-free paper
12 11 10 09 08 5 4 3 2 1
First Edition

Typeset in Adobe's AGaramond and Formata.

American Psychiatric Publishing, Inc.
1000 Wilson Boulevard
Arlington, VA 22209-3901
www.appi.org

Library of Congress Cataloging-in-Publication Data
Rothschild, Anthony J.
Clinical manual for diagnosis and treatment of psychotic depression / by Anthony J. Rothschild. — 1st ed.
p. ; cm.
Includes bibliographical references and index.
ISBN 978-1-58562-292-4 (alk. paper)
1. Psychotic depression—Diagnosis. 2. Psychotic depression—Treatment. I. Title. [DNLM: 1. Affective Disorders, Psychotic—diagnosis. 2. Affective Disorders, Psychotic—therapy. 3. Depressive Disorder—diagnosis. 4. Depressive Disorder—therapy. 5. Diagnosis, Differential. WM 207 R847c 2009]
RC537.R658 2009
616.85′27—dc22

2008037182

British Library Cataloguing in Publication Data
A CIP record is available from the British Library.

To Judy, Rachel, and Amanda;
my mother, Edith Rothschild;
and the memory of my father, Ernest Rothschild.

The book is also dedicated to Betty Brudnick
and in memory of Irving Brudnick,
without whose generous support
this book would not have been possible.

Contents

List of Tables and Figures

Preface

Periodically in newspapers across the globe, reporters tell a horrible story of a psychotically depressed woman who murders her children because she developed delusional beliefs regarding them. The case of Andrea Yates in Texas comes to mind. In 2001, Ms. Yates filled a bathtub with water and systematically drowned her five children. During her confession, she explained her actions by saying that she was not a good mother, the children were "not developing correctly," and she needed to be punished. Andrea Yates's illness is an example of psychotic depression, an illness with considerable morbidity and mortality.

A person with psychotic depression suffers from the dangerous combination of depressed mood and psychosis, with the psychosis commonly manifesting itself as nihilistic-type delusions (i.e., delusions that bad things are about to happen). Although psychotic depression is a very serious illness, it is treatable if properly diagnosed. Unfortunately, as I discuss in this book, the diagnosis is frequently missed, which can lead to the prescription of ineffective treatments, as well as unfortunate outcomes. Few clinicians have specialized in caring for patients with psychotic depression, and few psychiatric researchers have made the study of psychotic depression a priority. This lack of research interest is reflected in the fact that at the present time, no medications are approved by the U.S. Food and Drug Administration (FDA) for the treatment of psychotic depression, leaving clinicians to base their decisions regarding patient treatment on the very few studies that have been published in the medical literature.

Studies of treatments for psychotic depression have not been pursued because many clinicians and researchers, the pharmaceutical industry, and the National Institute of Mental Health (NIMH) have erroneously believed that psychotic depression is not a common illness. Nothing could be further from the truth. Based on studies in both inpatient and outpatient settings, an estimated 16%–54% of depressed adults are psychotic. Evidence indicates that the diagnosis is often missed in the emergency room and in inpatient hospital settings, leading to the misperception that the illness is not common (Rothschild et al. 2008). The lack of attention to developing treatments for psychotic depression is reflected not only by the fact that there are, as of this writing, no FDA-approved treatments for this disorder, but also by the fact that from 1983 to 2003 NIMH did not fund any studies of medication treatment for psychotic depression (Meyers et al. 2006). In addition, the second edition of the American Psychiatric Association's *Practice Guideline for the Treatment of Patients With Major Depressive Disorder* (2000) devotes only one paragraph to the treatment of psychotic depression.

Thus, I saw the need for this manual. I have spent more than 25 years in both clinical and research settings diagnosing and treating patients with psychotic depression and studying the diagnostic challenges, biology, course, and treatment of this serious disorder. I have attempted in this book to synthesize the published medical literature and my clinical experience into an easy-to-read, practical, evidence-based manual. I designed the book with the needs of the clinician, as well as the researcher-scientist, in mind, and I hope it will prove useful to psychiatrists, family and general practitioners, internists, neurologists, psychologists, nurses, social workers, and advanced students. More broadly, I hope that the book will be of interest to anyone seeking to learn more about the interplay of depression and psychosis that occurs in psychotic depression.

References

American Psychiatric Association: Practice Guideline for the Treatment of Patients With Major Depressive Disorder, 2nd Edition. Washington, DC, American Psychiatric Association, 2000

Meyers BS, Peasley-Miklus C, Flint AJ, et al: Methodological issues in designing a randomized controlled trial for psychotic depression: the STOP-PD Study. Psychiatr Ann 36:57–64, 2006

Rothschild AJ, Winer J, Flint AJ, et al; for the Study of Pharmacotherapy of Psychotic Depression (STOP-PD) Collaborative Study Group: Missed diagnosis of psychotic depression at 4 academic medical centers. J Clin Psychiatry 69:1293–1296, 2008

Disclosure of Competing Interests

Anthony J. Rothschild, M.D., has indicated a financial interest in or other affiliation with a commercial supporter, a manufacturer of a commercial product, a provider of a commercial service, a nongovernmental organization, and/or a government agency, as listed below:

Consultant: Forest Laboratories, Eli Lilly, Pfizer, and GlaxoSmithKline

Grant/research support: National Institute of Mental Health, Wyeth, Novartis, Cyberonics, Takeda

Eli Lilly and Pfizer provided study medication free of charge for the National Institute of Mental Health Study of the Pharmacotherapy of Psychotic Depression (STOP-PD)

Trademarks: The Rothschild Scale for Antidepressant Tachyphylaxis (RSAT); Rothschild Scale for Antidepressant Tachyphylaxis (RSAT)

Judith Shindul-Rothschild, Ph.D., R.N., C.S., has no competing interests during the year preceding manuscript submission to report.

Acknowledgments

I have many people to thank for their encouragement, advice, and support in preparing this book. My family has been patient and understanding of my need to spend time on this project. Irving and Betty Brudnick were instrumental by their endowment of the Irving S. and Betty Brudnick Endowed Chair at the University of Massachusetts Medical School, a position that has allowed me the time to focus on projects such as this manual. I am eternally indebted to Irving Brudnick's wisdom and support, and I miss his guidance greatly. At the American Psychiatric Press Inc., Robert Hales, Editor-in-Chief, John McDuffie, Editorial Director, and Greg Kuny, Managing Editor, deserve a great deal of credit for their unwavering confidence in me as an author and for their support throughout the development and production of this manual. My assistant Karen Lambert provided invaluable help in the typing of the manuscript, figures, and tables. I am grateful to have worked, during the National Institute of Mental Health Study of the Pharmacotherapy of Psychotic Depression (STOP-PD), with four outstanding clinician-scientists, each of whom is an expert on the diagnosis and treatment of psychotic depression: Alastair Flint, M.D., Barry Meyers, M.D., Benoit Mulsant, M.D., and Ellen Whyte, M.D. I am also appreciative of the support and encouragement of my colleagues and trainees at the University of Massachusetts Medical School and UMass Memorial Healthcare. Finally, this book could not have been written without the many patients and families with whom I have had the privilege of working.

1

Introduction

Psychotic depression—major depression with psychotic features, delusional depression—is a serious illness during which a person suffers from the dangerous combination of depressed mood and psychosis, with the psychosis commonly manifesting as nihilistic-type delusions (i.e., delusions that bad things are about to happen). Unfortunately, examples of psychotic depression are seen in the popular press in every part of the world: the mother who inexplicably kills her children before killing herself; the successful businessman who without warning jumps off a tall building; the retired, mild-mannered college professor who sets himself and his home on fire, killing all within. These are all real-life examples of psychotic depression—a serious, life-threatening illness. The great tragedy is that the illness is treatable if recognized. Unfortunately, as discussed in this manual, the diagnosis is frequently missed, leading to the prescription of ineffective treatments and to unfortunate outcomes.

The person with psychotic depression feels an unbearable horror, which greatly increases the risk of suicide for someone with this illness:

> Everything that occurs to the patient is interpreted in the light of the overmastering delusion. He feels himself universally despised and avoided; his sins are bruited abroad and are the subject of the contemptuous conversations of others; doctors and nurses draw aside their clothing to avoid infection as they pass his bed. Delusional ideas spring from the breeding-ground of a dominant anxiety: permanent breakdown of health, incapacity ever to work again, exclusion from all decent society, cancer, tuberculosis, death, damnation and hell stand like specters round the bed. It is hopeless to argue with the patients about these ideas; they cannot be convinced nor more than momentarily comforted, though sometimes they apparently welcome an opposition that permits an endless repetition of their ideas. (Slater and Roth 1969, p. 209)

Descriptions of psychotic depression can be found in ancient texts, including the Bible. In the book of Job, Job is depressed and feels that he has fallen from high status and has lost prestige. He has delusions of poverty and the nihilistic delusion that his children are dead, and he believes that he is giving off an unpleasant smell. He has the somatic delusion that he is covered from head to foot in boils—not a likely medical condition for him to have. His friends describe him as so changed that they hardly recognize him. In the book of Samuel, Saul, king of Israel, develops severe depression, guilt, and psychosis. During these episodes, he attempts to kill David and his son Jonathan, and later commits suicide himself.

It was not until the 1920s that any possible prognostic importance was attached to depressed patients having delusions. In 1921, Kraepelin noted that delusions in "manic-depressive insanity" were very frequent, particularly in the depressed state. The first attempt to study the prognostic importance of delusions in depressed patients was by Hoch and MacCurdy (1922), who examined whether outcome was influenced by the presence or absence of delusions. They suggested that absurd ideas in depressed patients predicted poor prognosis. However, the heterogeneity of their patient population makes it unclear what bearing their findings have in modern diagnostic terms (Glassman and Roose 1981). Similarly, in the early 1930s, various researchers (Anderson 1936; A.J. Lewis 1934a, 1934b, 1936; N.D.C. Lewis and Hubbard 1931; Steen 1933; Strecker et al. 1931) commented on the importance of delusions in the depressive syndrome, but lack of diagnostic clarity makes these reports difficult to interpret. Nonetheless, the studies are of interest for their clinical description of medication-free psychotic depressed patients.

In 1977, Kantor and Glassman reviewed the studies of A.J. Lewis (1934a, 1934b, 1936) using modern diagnostic criteria. They concluded, from the results of studies of delusional depression conducted prior to the introduction of electroconvulsive therapy (ECT), that 1) patients whose depression was accompanied by delusions generally did not do as well as nonpsychotic depressed patients; 2) the presence of delusions was not the sole predictor of outcome, because significant numbers of untreated patients with psychotic depression experienced complete symptom remission; and 3) the presence of delusions in patients with only a minimal mood disturbance was a poor prognostic sign.

By 1935, the introduction of ECT made the differentiation between psychotic and nonpsychotic depression less important because depressed patients had a good response to ECT whether or not delusions were present. Only patients with paranoid symptoms in the absence of a mood disorder did not respond favorably. With the introduction of tricyclic antidepressants and antipsychotic medications in the 1950s and 1960s, however, the differentiation between psychotic depression and nonpsychotic depression and between either type of depression and schizophrenia took on greater importance. Observations that psychotic depressed patients differed from nonpsychotic depressed patients in their response to pharmacologic treatments led investigators to focus on more clearly defining psychotic depression.

Professionals have long discussed whether psychotic depression is a distinct syndrome or simply represents a severe form of depression.

Much of the debate stems from the fact that in DSM-II (American Psychiatric Association 1968), *psychosis* referred to the severity of the depression and did not mean being out of touch with reality or having delusions or hallucinations. In 1970, Gerald Klerman, Eugene Paykel, and Brigitte Prusoff published an influential paper in which they stated that in depression there was a smooth continuum, without any demarcation points, from mild outpatient depression to severe depression requiring inpatient hospitalization (Paykel et al. 1970).

In 1992, as DSM-IV was being planned, Schatzberg and Rothschild (1992) made a strong argument in the *American Journal of Psychiatry* that there was sufficient evidence at that time, from studies of clinical characteristics and symptoms, biology, family history, course and outcome, and treatment, that psychotic depression should be a distinct illness in DSM-IV, separate from major depression. Besides presenting the scientific rationale, they indicated that if psychotic depression had its own diagnostic category, it would increase awareness of the disorder among clinicians, who often missed the diagnosis. They also hoped that the pharmaceutical industry and the National Institute of Mental Health, both of which had not been paying much attention to this disorder, would devote more resources to study effective treatments for psychotic depression.

The *American Journal of Psychiatry* article led to a position paper submitted to the DSM-IV Work Group on Mood Disorders (Schatzberg and Rothschild 1996). The work group agreed (Schatzberg and Rothschild 1996) that the clinical relevance of specifically designating patients as having psychotic depression was high, and the work group considered two options: 1) to continue the classification as in DSM-III-R (American Psychiatric Association 1987), by designating psychosis as a decimal point under the severity code; or 2) to designate psychotic depression as a separate syndrome, "major depression with psychotic features." The work group argued that the advantage of option 1 was that it ensured that psychotic depression had a specific numerical code. The disadvantage was that it still implied that psychosis was at the end of a severity continuum, which option 2 did not imply. However, the work group then argued that if option 2 were selected

> for administrative reasons, the syndrome might not receive its own numerical code, which would then limit the practicality of any such designation, and the crosswalk to ICD-10 would be made impractical. After much deliberation, the Work Group recommended the first option, although it recognized it was less than optimal. (Schatzberg and Rothschild 1996, pp. 173–174)

Thus, in DSM-IV (American Psychiatric Association 1994) and DSM-IV-TR (American Psychiatric Association 2000a), psychotic depression remains a subclassification of major depression. To receive the diagnosis, a patient must first meet the criteria for major depression (see Table 1–1), for which the first three diagnosis digits are 296. The fourth digit (the digit after the decimal point) is either 2 (if it is the patient's first episode) or 3 (if it is a recurrent episode). Then, if the patient exhibits psychotic symptoms (either delusions or hallucinations), the fifth digit is 4, indicating "severe with psychotic features" (American Psychiatric Association 2000a) (see Table 1–2).

One can see in this classification the historical remnants of the DSM-II interpretation of *psychosis* as meaning "severe." Thus, in both DSM-IV and DSM-IV-TR, psychotic depression has remained as a subclassification—that is, a specifier—of major depression on the continuum of severity. Table 1–3 lists the five possible DSM codes for a patient with psychotic depression.

Because psychotic depression has been ignored as a distinct illness, despite its significant morbidity and mortality, very few psychiatric researchers have made the study of psychotic depression a priority, and the diagnosis is frequently missed by clinicians (Rothschild et al. 2008). Sadly, at present, no medications have been approved by the U.S. Food and Drug Administration for the treatment of psychotic depression. This lack of approved medications is due in part to the pharmaceutical industry's lack of interest in developing medications for the treatment

Table 1–1. DSM-IV-TR criteria for major depressive episode

A. Five (or more) of the following symptoms have been present during the same 2-week period and represent a change from previous functioning; at least one of the symptoms is either (1) depressed mood or (2) loss of interest or pleasure.

Note: Do not include symptoms that are clearly due to a general medical condition, or mood-incongruent delusions or hallucinations.

(1) depressed mood most of the day, nearly every day, as indicated by either subjective report (e.g., feels sad or empty) or observation made by others (e.g., appears tearful). **Note:** In children and adolescents, can be irritable mood.

(2) markedly diminished interest or pleasure in all, or almost all, activities most of the day, nearly every day (as indicated by either subjective account or observation made by others)

(3) significant weight loss when not dieting or weight gain (e.g., a change of more than 5% of body weight in a month), or decrease or increase in appetite nearly every day. **Note:** In children, consider failure to make expected weight gains.

(4) insomnia or hypersomnia nearly every day

(5) psychomotor agitation or retardation nearly every day (observable by others, not merely subjective feelings of restlessness or being slowed down)

(6) fatigue or loss of energy nearly every day

(7) feelings of worthlessness or excessive or inappropriate guilt (which may be delusional) nearly every day (not merely self-reproach or guilt about being sick)

(8) diminished ability to think or concentrate, or indecisiveness, nearly every day (either by subjective account or as observed by others)

(9) recurrent thoughts of death (not just fear of dying), recurrent suicidal ideation without a specific plan, or a suicide attempt or a specific plan for committing suicide

Table 1–1. DSM-IV-TR criteria for major depressive episode *(continued)*

B. The symptoms do not meet criteria for a mixed episode.

C. The symptoms cause clinically significant distress or impairment in social, occupational, or other important areas of functioning.

D. The symptoms are not due to the direct physiological effects of a substance (e.g., a drug of abuse, a medication) or a general medical condition (e.g., hypothyroidism).

E. The symptoms are not better accounted for by bereavement, i.e., after the loss of a loved one, the symptoms persist for longer than 2 months or are characterized by marked functional impairment, morbid preoccupation with worthlessness, suicidal ideation, psychotic symptoms, or psychomotor retardation.

Source. Reprinted from *Diagnostic and Statistical Manual of Mental Disorders,* 4th Edition, Text Revision. Washington, DC, American Psychiatric Association, 2000. p. 356. Copyright 2000, American Psychiatric Association. Used with permission.

of psychotic depression.[1] Antidepressants are first developed and studied for the treatment of nonpsychotic depression, and patients with psychotic depression are excluded from participating. Similarly, antipsychotic medications are developed first for the treatment of schizophrenia and schizoaffective disorder, then for bipolar mania, and are not studied in patients with psychotic depression. Consequently, the clinician is forced to extrapolate from studies of antidepressant and antipsychotic medications for illnesses other than psychotic depression.

Studies of treatments for psychotic depression also have not been pursued because, in my opinion, the business side of the pharmaceutical industry wrongly believes that patients with psychotic depression do not represent a "big market." As discussed in Chapter 2, "Epidemiology," psychotic depression is a more common illness than is generally realized;

[1]There is one exception: Eli Lilly and Company studied the combination of olanzapine and fluoxetine (see Rothschild et al. 2004).

Table 1–2. DSM-IV-TR criteria for severity/psychotic/remission specifiers for current (or most recent) major depressive episode

Note: Code in fifth digit. Mild, moderate, severe without psychotic features, and severe with psychotic features can be applied only if the criteria are currently met for a major depressive episode. In partial remission and in full remission can be applied to the most recent major depressive episode in major depressive disorder and to a major depressive episode in bipolar I or II disorder only if it is the most recent type of mood episode.

.x1—**Mild:** Few, if any, symptoms in excess of those required to make the diagnosis and symptoms result in only minor impairment in occupational functioning or in usual social activities or relationships with others.

.x2—**Moderate:** Symptoms or functional impairment between "mild" and "severe."

.x3—**Severe without psychotic features:** Several symptoms in excess of those required to make the diagnosis, **and** symptoms markedly interfere with occupational functioning or with usual social activities or relationships with others.

.x4—**Severe with psychotic features:** Delusions or hallucinations. If possible, specify whether the psychotic features are mood-congruent or mood-incongruent:

> **Mood-congruent psychotic features:** Delusions or hallucinations whose content is entirely consistent with the typical depressive themes of personal inadequacy, guilt, disease, death, nihilism, or deserved punishment.
>
> **Mood-incongruent psychotic features:** Delusions or hallucinations whose content does not involve typical depressive themes of personal inadequacy, guilt, disease, death, nihilism, or deserved punishment. Included are such symptoms as persecutory delusions (not directly related to depressive themes), thought insertion, thought broadcasting, and delusions of control.

Table 1–2. DSM-IV-TR criteria for severity/psychotic/remission specifiers for current (or most recent) major depressive episode *(continued)*

.x5—In partial remission: Symptoms of a major depressive episode are present but full criteria are not met, or there is a period without any significant symptoms of a major depressive episode lasting less than 2 months following the end of the major depressive episode. (If the major depressive episode was superimposed on dysthymic disorder, the diagnosis of dysthymic disorder alone is given once the full criteria for a major depressive episode are no longer met.)

.x6—In full remission: During the past 2 months, no significant signs or symptoms of the disturbance were present.

.x0—Unspecified.

Source. Reprinted from *Diagnostic and Statistical Manual of Mental Disorders,* 4th Edition, Text Revision. Washington, DC, American Psychiatric Association, 2000, p. 413. Copyright 2000, American Psychiatric Association. Used with permission.

on the basis of studies done in both inpatient and outpatient settings, an estimated 16%–54% of depressed adults have psychosis. Unfortunately, evidence indicates that the diagnosis of psychotic depression is often missed in the emergency room and inpatient hospital settings (see Chapter 5, "Diagnosis and Assessment"), which leads to the misperception that the illness is not common.

Developing treatments for psychotic depression not only has been ignored by the pharmaceutical industry but also has received little attention from scientific granting agencies of the U.S. government and in publications of practice guidelines. Although psychotic depression is a significant public health problem, from 1983 to 2003 the National Institute of Mental Health did not fund any studies of the medication treatment of psychotic depression (Meyers et al. 2006). Furthermore, the American Psychiatric Association's (2000b) *Practice Guideline for the Treatment of Patients With Major Depressive Disorder* devotes only one paragraph to the treatment of psychotic depression.

Table 1–3. DSM-IV-TR diagnostic codes for psychotic depression

296.24	Major depressive disorder, single episode, severe with psychotic features
296.34	Major depressive disorder, recurrent, severe with psychotic features
296.44	Bipolar I disorder, most recent episode manic, severe with psychotic features
296.54	Bipolar I disorder, most recent episode depressed, severe with psychotic features
296.64	Bipolar I disorder, most recent episode mixed, severe with psychotic features

The purpose of this manual is to provide the reader with state-of-the-art information on the epidemiology, genetics/family history, and diagnosis of psychotic depression. It also is intended to serve as a practical guide for the individual assessment and treatment of the patient who suffers from psychotic depression.

In Chapter 2 ("Epidemiology"), I discuss the prevalence of psychotic depression in the community and in different clinical settings. Chapter 3 ("Family Studies and Genetics") reviews the rates of psychiatric illness in families of patients with psychotic depression as well as the genes hypothesized to play a role in psychotic depression. In Chapter 4 ("Biology"), I review studies of the hypothalamic-pituitary-adrenal axis, dopaminergic and serotonergic systems, growth hormone, and neuroimaging in patients with psychotic depression. Chapter 5 ("Diagnosis and Assessment") summarizes the challenges and difficulties in assessing and accurately diagnosing psychotic depression. In Chapter 6 ("Treatment"), I discuss the evidence base for the treatment of psychotic depression and provide practical advice for treating psychotic depression with medication, ECT, and psychotherapy. Chapter 7

("Course and Cognition") reviews the course of psychotic depression, as well as the cognitive problems (in addition to psychosis) that are frequently observed in patients with this condition. In Chapter 8 ("Treatment Settings") I review the variety of settings—outpatient, partial hospitalization, day treatment, and inpatient—in which the treatment of patients with psychotic depression occurs. Chapter 9 ("Nursing Care") focuses on the important role of nursing case in the assessment and management of patients with psychotic depression. The manual concludes, in Chapter 10 ("Special Populations and Issues"), with a discussion of suicide risk in patients with psychotic depression. I also discuss the presentation and treatment of the disorder in special populations, including women in the postpartum, children and adolescents, and older adults.

Key Clinical Points

- Psychotic depression has been described throughout recorded history.
- Psychotic depression is more common than is generally realized.
- There has been a debate as to whether psychotic depression is a distinct syndrome or a severe form of depression.
- The diagnosis of psychotic depression is frequently missed by clinicians.
- The U.S. Food and Drug Administration has not approved any medications for the treatment of psychotic depression.

References

American Psychiatric Association: Diagnostic and Statistical Manual of Mental Disorders, 2nd Edition. Washington, DC, American Psychiatric Association, 1968

American Psychiatric Association: Diagnostic and Statistical Manual of Mental Disorders, 3rd Edition, Revised. Washington, DC, American Psychiatric Association, 1987

American Psychiatric Association: Diagnostic and Statistical Manual of Mental Disorders, 4th Edition. Washington, DC, American Psychiatric Association, 1994

American Psychiatric Association: Diagnostic and Statistical Manual of Mental Disorders, 4th Edition, Text Revision. Washington, DC, American Psychiatric Association, 2000a

American Psychiatric Association: Practice Guideline for the Treatment of Patients With Major Depressive Disorder, 2nd Edition. Washington, DC, American Psychiatric Association, 2000b

Anderson EW: Prognosis of the depressions of later life. J Ment Sci 82:559–588, 1936

Glassman AH, Roose SP: Delusional depression: a distinct clinical entity? Arch Gen Psychiatry 38:424–427, 1981

Hoch A, MacCurdy JT: The prognosis of involutional melancholia. Arch Neurol Psychiatry 7:1–17, 1922

Kantor SJ, Glassman AH: Delusional depressions: natural history and response to treatment. Br J Psychiatry 131:351–360, 1977

Kraepelin E: Manic-Depressive Insanity and Paranoia. Translated by Barclay RM. Edinburgh, UK, E & S Livingstone, 1921

Lewis AJ: Melancholia: a clinical survey of depressive states. J Ment Sci 80:277–378, 1934a

Lewis AJ: Melancholia: a historical review. J Ment Sci 80:1–42, 1934b

Lewis AJ: Melancholia: prognostic study and case material. J Ment Sci 82:488–558, 1936

Lewis NDC, Hubbard LD: The mechanisms and prognostic aspects of manic-depressive-schizophrenic combinations. Proceedings of the Association for Research in Nervous and Mental Diseases 11:539–610, 1931

Meyers BS, Peasley-Miklus C, Flint AJ, et al: Methodological issues in designing a randomized controlled trial for psychotic depression: the STOP-PD study. Psychiatr Ann 36:57–64, 2006

Paykel ES, Klerman GL, Prusoff B: Treatment setting and clinical depression. Arch Gen Psychiatry 22:11–21, 1970

Rothschild AJ, Williamson DJ, Tohen MF, et al: A double-blind, randomized study of olanzapine and olanzapine/fluoxetine combination for major depression with psychotic features. J Clin Psychopharmacol 24:365–373, 2004

Rothschild AJ, Winer J, Flint AJ, et al; for the Study of Pharmacotherapy of Psychotic Depression (STOP-PD) Collaborative Study Group: Missed diagnosis of psychotic depression at 4 academic medical centers. J Clin Psychiatry 69:1293–1296, 2008

Schatzberg AF, Rothschild AJ: Psychotic (delusional) major depression: should it be included as a distinct syndrome in DSM-IV? Am J Psychiatry 149:733–745, 1992

Schatzberg AF, Rothschild AJ: Psychotic (delusional) major depression: should it be included as a distinct syndrome in DSM-IV? in DSM-IV Sourcebook, Vol 2. Edited by Widiger TA, Frances AJ, Pincus HA, et al. Washington, DC, American Psychiatric Press, 1996, pp 127–180

Slater E, Roth M: Clinical Psychiatry, 3rd Edition. London, Baillière, Tindall & Cassel, 1969

Steen RB: Prognosis in manic-depressive psychoses. Psychiatr Q 7:419–429, 1933

Strecker EA, Appel KE, Eyman EV, et al: The prognosis in manic-depressive psychosis. Proceedings of the Association for Research in Nervous and Mental Diseases 11:471–537, 1931

Recommended Reading

Glassman AH, Roose SP: Delusional depression: a distinct clinical entity? Arch Gen Psychiatry 38:424–427, 1981

Schatzberg AF, Rothschild AJ: Psychotic (delusional) major depression: should it be included as a distinct syndrome in DSM-IV? Am J Psychiatry 149:733–745, 1992

Schatzberg AF, Rothschild AJ: Psychotic (delusional) major depression: should it be included as a distinct syndrome in DSM-IV? in DSM-IV Sourcebook, Vol 2. Edited by Widiger TA, Frances AJ, Pincus HA, et al. Washington, DC, American Psychiatric Press, 1996, pp 127–180

2

Epidemiology

Prevalence of Psychotic Depression in the Community

The lifetime prevalence rate of psychotic depression varies depending on the setting (see Table 2–1). Epidemiological studies of the prevalence of psychotic depression in the community indicate that approximately 4 per 1,000 people in the general population have the illness, although the community rates in people over age 60 have been reported to be 14–30 per 1,000 (Baldwin and Jolley 1986; Blazer 1994).

For example, Perälä et al. (2007) screened a nationally representative sample of 8,028 persons age 30 years or older for psychotic and bipolar I disorders, using the Composite International Diagnostic Interview, self-reported diagnoses, medical examination, and national registers, and interviewed with the Structured Clinical Interview for DSM-IV. They found that 0.35% of the people in the community met criteria for unipolar psychotic depression. In people age 65 years or older, the rate of psy-

Table 2–1. Prevalence rates of psychotic depression

Population	Rate
Community samples	0.4%
Community samples (elderly)	0.43%–3.0%
Major depression (community)	14.7%–18.5%
Major depression (outpatient adolescents)	18%
Major depression (inpatients)	25%
Major depression (elderly inpatients)	24%–53%
Major depression (adolescent inpatients)	45%

chotic depression was 0.43% (Perälä et al. 2007). In another study, of 18,980 people ages 15–100 years who were representative of the general populations of several European countries, the prevalence of psychotic depression was 4 per 1,000 people (Ohayon and Schatzberg 2002).

Among persons over age 60, the prevalence of psychotic depression in the community is even higher, between 14 and 30 per 1,000 (Baldwin and Jolley 1986; Blazer 1994). In a Finnish community sample of people over age 60, the rate of psychotic depression was 12 per 1,000 women and 6 per 1,000 men (Kivela and Pahkala 1989).

Patients With Major Depression

In samples of patients with major depression, the rates of psychotic depression are considerably higher than in the general community population. In a European study, 18.5% of patients who met the criteria for major depression also fulfilled the criteria for major depressive episode with psychotic features (Ohayon and Schatzberg 2002). In the United States, results from the Epidemiologic Catchment Area study (Johnson et al. 1991) indicated that 14.7% of patients who met the criteria for major depression had a history of psychotic features. In outpatient studies of adolescents with major depression, the prevalence of psychotic symptoms was reported to be 18% (Ryan et al. 1987).

Prevalence of Psychotic Depression in the Inpatient Setting

In studies of patients with major depression in an inpatient setting, the prevalence rate of psychotic depression is even higher than in patients with major depression in the community. In a study of consecutively admitted patients hospitalized for major depression, Coryell and colleagues (1984) reported that 25% of the patients met criteria for psychotic depression. In samples of older inpatients with major depression, the prevalence of psychotic depression increases dramatically. Studies have reported that in inpatient settings, 24%–53% of people older than 60 who have major depression have psychotic depression (Gournellis and Lykouras 2006; Meyers and Greenberg 1986). In an inpatient sample of depressed adolescents, 45% of the adolescents had psychotic features (Haley et al. 1988).

Prevalence of Psychotic Depression in Patients With Unipolar Versus Bipolar Disorder

Table 2–2 summarizes findings of studies that examined the prevalence of psychotic features in patients with unipolar or bipolar depression. As shown in the table, psychotic features are significantly more common in bipolar depressed patients than in unipolar depressed patients (χ^2=54.39, df=1, $P \leq 0.001$). These results are interesting in light of other studies that indicate that when a patient with bipolar disorder gets depressed, the depressed episode is likely to be an episode with psychotic features (see Chapter 5, "Diagnosis and Assessment").

As shown in Table 2–2, studies published between 1971 and 1984 largely failed to support a difference between patients with unipolar and

Table 2–2. Psychotic depression in unipolar and bipolar patients

Study	Diagnoses (*n*)	Proportion of patients with delusions and/or hallucinations	Comments
Beigel and Murphy 1971	25 BP 25 UP	BP: 12% UP: 36%	Not statistically significant Patients matched for age, sex, and level of depression Bipolar patients required to have had manic episode on ward; thus, 34 bipolar patients excluded from study
Guze et al. 1975	19 BP 139 UP	BP: 53% UP: 17%	$P<0.01$ Phase of bipolar illness unclear
Kathol and Winokur 1977[a]	32 BP 561 UP	BP: 41% UP: 31%	Not statistically significant
Winokur 1984	122 BP 203 UP **Feighner et al. criteria**	BP: 64% UP: 56%	Not statistically significant Phase not specified Auditory and visual hallucinations more likely in BP than in UP

Table 2–2. Psychotic depression in unipolar and bipolar patients *(continued)*

Study	Diagnoses (*n*)	Proportion of patients with delusions and/or hallucinations	Comments
Endicott et al. 1985	122 BP 104 UP (recurrent) **RDC**	BP: 29%,[b] 22%[c] UP: 14%,[b] 11%[c]	Not statistically significant BP>UP among female subgroups (P<0.05)
Andreasen et al. 1988	177 BP 422 UP		Tendency for greater severity of psychotic symptoms, particularly delusional thinking, in BP
Black and Nasrallah 1989	161 BP 763 UP **DSM-III criteria**	BP: 16.8% UP: 18.6%	No probability value reported Retrospective case note review
Thakur et al. 1999	86 BP 588 UP **DSM-III criteria**	BP: 39.5% UP: 26.4%	Tendency (P=0.09, OR=1.51) for PD to be associated with BP diagnosis compared with NPD

Table 2–2. Psychotic depression in unipolar and bipolar patients *(continued)*

Study	Diagnoses (*n*)	Proportion of patients with delusions and/or hallucinations	Comments
Parker et al. 2000	83 BP 904 UP **DSM-III/III-R criteria**	BP: 19.3%,[d] 19.3%[e] UP: 10.4%,[d] 9.7%[e]	OR=2.05 (DSM-III/III-R diagnosis) and 2.21 ("clinical" diagnosis) Consolidated three databases Used DSM-III/III-R, clinical, and "CORE" subtyping systems BP patients more likely to receive diagnosis of melancholia and of PD
Mitchell et al. 2001	39 BP 39 UP **DSM-IV criteria**	BP: 38.7%[f] UP: 10.3%[f]	BP>UP, $P<0.05$ Matched for gender, age, and presence of melancholic subtype

Note. BP=bipolar disorder; NPD=nonpsychotic depression; OR=odds ratio; PD=psychotic depression; RDC=Research Diagnostic Criteria; UP=unipolar disorder.

[a]Combined data set from Winokur and Clayton 1967 and Winokur 1975. [b]Lifetime diagnosis. [c]Intake episode involving PD. [d]DSM-III diagnoses. [e]"Clinical" diagnosis according to preestablished criteria of Parker et al. 1990. [f]In previous depressive episodes.

bipolar illness in the frequency of hallucinations and delusions during depression (Beigel and Murphy 1971; Kathol and Winokur 1977; Winokur 1984). The exception was the study by Guze and colleagues (1975), who reported that psychotic features were more frequent among bipolar patients (53%) than among primary unipolar patients (17%) ($P<0.01$). However, the authors did not report whether these patients were in the manic or depressed phase of the illness. Beigel and Murphy (1971) did not find a relationship between psychotic depression and polarity, in part because psychosis itself was a criterion for inclusion in the study. Furthermore, the sample size was small and unusual in that patients were required to have displayed a manic episode while on the research ward; thus, 34 bipolar patients were excluded. Finally, the investigators relied on assessment of behavior rather than direct patient interview, which may have resulted in underreporting of symptoms. Kathol and Winokur (1977) combined four separate data sets and found no clear difference in the percentages of bipolar versus unipolar depressed patients with hallucinations or delusions. These combined data should, however, be viewed cautiously because they are retrospective in nature and represent different study populations evaluated by different investigators under nonuniform conditions.

More recent and better-designed studies have generally observed a relationship between psychotic depression and polarity (Endicott et al. 1985; Mitchell et al. 2001; Parker et al. 2000; Thakur et al. 1999), with psychotic depression more commonly observed in bipolar depressed patients than in unipolar depressed patients. However, not all studies are in agreement (Black and Nasrallah 1989).

Key Clinical Points

- The prevalence of psychotic depression in the community is approximately 4 per 1,000.
- Community prevalence of psychotic depression is higher in older adults (4–30 per 1,000).

- The prevalence of psychotic depression is highest among inpatients with the diagnosis of major depression (25%–53%).
- In adolescents, the prevalence of psychotic depression ranges from 18% (outpatients) to 45% (inpatients).
- Psychotic depression appears to be prevalent in patients with bipolar disorder.

References

Andreasen NC, Endicott J, Coryell W, et al: The phenomenology of bipolar depression, in 1988 New Research Program and Abstracts, American Psychiatric Association 141st Annual Meeting, Montreal, Quebec, Canada, May 7–12, 1988. Washington, DC, American Psychiatric Association, 1988

Baldwin RC, Jolley DJ: The prognosis of depression in old age. Br J Psychiatry 149:574–583, 1986

Beigel A, Murphy D: Unipolar and bipolar affective illness: differences in clinical characteristics accompanying depression. Arch Gen Psychiatry 24:215–220, 1971

Black DW, Nasrallah A: Hallucinations and delusions in 1,715 patients with unipolar and bipolar affective disorders. Psychopathology 22:28–34, 1989

Blazer D: Epidemiology of late-life depression, in Diagnosis and Treatment of Depression in Late Life. Edited by Schneider L, Reynolds C, Lebowitz B, et al. Washington, DC, American Psychiatric Press, 1994, pp 9–20

Coryell W, Pfohl B, Zimmerman M: The clinical and neuroendocrine features of psychotic depression. J Nerv Ment Dis 172:521–528, 1984

Endicott J, Nee J, Andreasen N, et al: Bipolar II: combine or keep separate? J Affect Disord 8:17–28, 1985

Gournellis R, Lykouras L: Psychotic (delusional) major depression in the elderly: a review. Curr Psychiatry Rev 2:235–244, 2006

Guze A, Woodruff R, Clayton P: The significance of psychotic affective disorders. Arch Gen Psychiatry 32:1147–1150, 1975

Haley GMT, Fine S, Marriage K: Psychotic features in adolescents with major depression. J Am Acad Child Adolesc Psychiatry 27:489–493, 1988

Johnson J, Horwath E, Weissman MM: The validity of major depression with psychotic features based on a community sample. Arch Gen Psychiatry 48:1075–1081, 1991

Kathol R, Winokur G: "Organic" and "psychotic" symptoms in unipolar (UP) vs bipolar (BP) depressions. Compr Psychiatry 18:251–253, 1977

Kivela SL, Pahkala K: Delusional depression in the elderly: a community study. Z Gerontol 22:236–241, 1989

Meyers BS, Greenberg R: Late-life delusional depression. J Affect Disord 11:133–137, 1986

Mitchell PB, Wilhelm K, Parker G, et al: The clinical features of bipolar depression: a comparison with matched major depressive disorder patients. J Clin Psychiatry 62:212–216, 2001

Ohayon MM, Schatzberg AF: Prevalence of depressive episodes with psychotic features in the general population. Am J Psychiatry 159:1855–1861, 2002

Parker G, Hadzi-Pavlovic D, Boyce P, et al: Classifying depression by mental state signs. Br J Psychiatry 157:55–65, 1990

Parker G, Roy K, Wilhelm K, et al: The nature of bipolar depression: implications for the definition of melancholia. J Affect Disord 59:217–224, 2000

Perälä J, Suvisaari J, Saarni SI, et al: Lifetime prevalence of psychotic and bipolar I disorders in a general population. Arch Gen Psychiatry 64:19–28, 2007

Ryan ND, Puig-Antich J, Ambrosini P, et al: The clinical picture of major depression in children and adolescents. Arch Gen Psychiatry 44:854–861, 1987

Thakur M, Hays J, Krishnan RR: Clinical, demographic and social characteristics of psychotic depression. Psychiatry Res 86:99–106, 1999

Winokur G: The Iowa 500: heterogeneity and course in manic-depressive illness (bipolar). Compr Psychiatry 16:125–131, 1975

Winokur G, Clayton PJ: Family history studies, I: two types of affective disorders separated according to genetic and clinical factors, in Recent Advances in Biological Psychiatry, Vol 9. Edited by Wortis J. New York, Plenum, 1967

Winokur G: Psychosis in bipolar and unipolar affective illness with special reference to schizo-affective disorder. Br J Psychiatry 145:236–242, 1984

Recommended Reading

Johnson J, Horwath E, Weissman MM: The validity of major depression with psychotic features based on a community sample. Arch Gen Psychiatry 48:1075–1081, 1991

Ohayon MM, Schatzberg AF: Prevalence of depressive episodes with psychotic features in the general population. Am J Psychiatry 159:1855–1861, 2002

Perälä J, Suvisaari J, Saarni SI, et al: Lifetime prevalence of psychotic and bipolar I disorders in a general population. Arch Gen Psychiatry 64:19–28, 2007

3

Family Studies and Genetics

Family Studies

The families of people who have psychotic depression may show a greater prevalence of psychotic depression, bipolar disorder, and depression in general than the families of people who have nonpsychotic depression (see Table 3–1). However, not all studies are in agreement (Bond et al. 1986; Coryell and Tsuang 1982; Coryell et al. 1984; Frangos et al. 1983; Leckman et al. 1984; Maj et al. 1991; Nelson et al. 1984; Price et al. 1984; Weissman et al. 1984, 1988).

Prevalence of Psychotic Depression

In a large family study of major depression (Leckman et al. 1984), the first-degree relatives of patients with psychotic depression showed a high rate (10.3%) of psychotic depression. In addition, of the depressed

Table 3–1. Studies of families of individuals with psychotic depression

↑ Psychotic depression
↑ Bipolar disorder
↑ Depression in general

first-degree relatives of patients with psychotic depression, 37% also had psychotic features, providing some evidence that psychotic depression "breeds true within the affected families" (Leckman et al. 1984, p. 837).

Prevalence of Bipolar Disorder

Weissman and colleagues (1984), in a family study of major depression, found the prevalence of bipolar illness to be nearly six times as high among the relatives of probands with psychotic depression as among the relatives of probands with nonpsychotic depression or among the relatives of control subjects, although this has not been observed in other studies (Coryell et al. 1984; Price et al. 1984). Subsequently, Weissman and colleagues (1988) presented data derived from a direct-interview study of 220 offspring (ages 6–23 years) of probands with psychotic major depression, probands with nonpsychotic major depression, and psychiatrically healthy controls. The children of psychotic probands had nearly a threefold increase in cyclothymia when compared with the children of nonpsychotic probands. The authors concluded that because there is general agreement that cyclothymia is related to bipolar disorder, their data suggest a relationship between the psychotic subtype of major depression and bipolar spectrum disorders.

Endicott and colleagues (1986) studied the lifetime diagnoses of first-degree relatives of patients hospitalized with Research Diagnostic Criteria–diagnosed schizoaffective disorder, depressed subtype; major depressive disorder, psychotic subtype; or major depressive disorder, nonpsychotic subtype. They found that 10% of patients with psychotic depression had at least one directly interviewed first-degree relative with bipolar disorder, psychotic subtype, compared with only 2.6% of patients with nonpsychotic major depressive disorder (relative risk=3.69, $P<0.05$). Blacker and colleagues (1996) found that unipolar relatives of bipolar probands were more likely to have more severe, even psychotic, depression than were unipolar relatives of control subjects (20% vs. 5%, respectively; $P=0.04$).

Prevalence of Major Depression, Nonpsychotic

In some studies, the first-degree relatives of patients with psychotic depression exhibit higher rates of depression in general (Leckman et al. 1984; Nelson et al. 1984) than the family members of patients with nonpsychotic depression. In one study (Bond et al. 1986) using the dexamethasone suppression test, when patients with psychotic depression were divided by degree of hypothalamic-pituitary-adrenal axis dysregulation, the prevalence of depression was significantly higher in the first-degree relatives of probands with psychotic depression with high postdexamethasone cortisol levels (>15 µg/dL) than in the first-degree relatives of probands with low or intermediate postdexamethasone cortisol levels (0–14.9 µg/dL).

Genetics

Several genes have been identified as candidates for possible involvement in psychotic depression (see Table 3–2). Unfortunately, most studies to date that have examined the involvement of these specific genes in psychotic depression have yielded negative results.

Dopamine-β-Hydroxylase Gene

Patients with psychotic depression have low activity of dopamine-β-hydroxylase (DBH), the key enzyme that converts dopamine to norepinephrine (Meltzer et al. 1976; Meyers et al. 1999; Mod et al. 1986; Sapru et al. 1989). This enzyme has been hypothesized to play an impor-

Table 3–2. Gene candidates for psychotic depression

Dopamine-β-hydroxylase gene (adenosine allele)
Serotonin transporter gene; 5-HT_{1A}, 5-HT_{2A}, 5-HT_{2C} receptor genes
Dopamine D_4 receptor gene (*DRD4* allele 7)
Glycogen synthase kinase–3 gene (beta isoform)

tant role in why some depressed patients become psychotic (Schatzberg et al. 1985) (see Chapter 4, "Biology"). DBH deficiency is associated with a lower dopamine-to-norepinephrine ratio (Robertson et al. 1991). The gene encoding DBH is located on chromosome 9q34 (Craig et al. 1988) and appears to be a major quantitative trait locus controlling serum and cerebrospinal fluid DBH activity (Cubells et al. 1998; Wei et al. 1997, 1998; Wilson et al. 1988; Zabetian et al. 2001). Consequently, research into a genetic basis for psychotic depression has started with the genes involved in controlling DBH activity.

Wood and colleagues (2002) suggested that the presence of the A (adenosine) allele of the DBH gene in depressed patients may confer an independently inherited vulnerability to psychosis and that the GG (guanine, guanine) genotype may protect against the development of psychosis. The GG genotype is associated with higher DBH activity, and hence lower dopamine levels, which may be a key protective mechanism against psychosis vulnerability (see Chapter 4, "Biology").

A study by Cubells and colleagues (2002), which replicated the lower DBH activity in psychotic depression than in nonpsychotic depression, could not account for the lower plasma levels of DBH in patients with psychotic depression by DBH genotype. The authors hypothesized that other variants at the DBH gene locus, or at other loci, might account for the findings.

Serotonergic and Dopaminergic System Genes

One group of researchers has reported that none of the serotonergic system candidate genes they examined (polymorphisms in the genes for the serotonin [5-HT] transporter and 5-HT_{1A}, 5-HT_{2A}, and 5-HT_{2C} receptors) appeared to be involved in psychotic depression (Serretti et al. 1999a, 1999c, 2000). However, long variants of the dopamine D_4 gene *(DRD4)* allele 7, which is associated with reduced cAMP (cyclic adenosine monophosphate) formation, were found to be statistically significantly associated with scores on the delusional subscale of the Hamilton Rating Scale for Depression in a combined sample of patients with bipolar or unipolar depression, as well as for unipolar depressed patients and bipolar depressed patients analyzed separately (Serretti et al. 1998). This same group found *DRD4* variants (specifically, the exon 3 allele 7 variant vs. allele 2) to be associated with delusional symptoms among a mixed group of 461 patients with major psychoses (Serretti et al. 1999d), but subsequently reported that in a larger group, *DRD4* variants did not appear to play a major role in risk for psychosis (Serretti et al. 1999b). Short alleles, rather than longer alleles, are associated with unipolar depression and bipolar disorder (Serretti et al. 1999d).

Glycogen Synthase Kinase–3 Gene

Other genetic studies have focused on the glycogen synthase kinase–3 (GSK-3) enzyme, a proline-directed serine-threonine kinase that was initially identified as a phosphorylating and inactivating glycogen synthase, which is critical in the regulation of glucose storage (Embi et al. 1980). The two isoforms that exist, α and β, show a high degree of amino acid homology (Stambolic and Woodgett 1994). GSK-3β is inhibited by lithium (Klein and Melton 1996), and this effect has been hypothesized to underlie lithium's efficacy in mood disorders (Detera-Wadleigh 2001; Manji et al. 2000; Salinas and Hall 1999). Some studies have observed an association between GSK-3β and both psychotic and personality features in patients with mood disorder (Serretti et al. 2008), suggesting that neurodegenerative processes linked to GSK-3β may in part be responsible for delusional symptoms and specific personality dimensions in these patients.

Key Clinical Points

- Few genetic studies exist of families in which the probands have psychotic depression.
- Families of probands with psychotic depression exhibit a higher prevalence of psychotic depression, bipolar disorder, and nonpsychotic depression.
- First-degree relatives of patients with psychotic depression have a high rate (10.3%) of psychotic depression.
- Thirty-seven percent of first-degree relatives of patients with psychotic depression exhibit psychotic features.
- Several genes (e.g., dopamine-β-hydroxylase gene, dopamine D_4 receptor gene [allele 7]) have been proposed to play a role in psychotic depression.

References

Blacker D, Faraone SV, Rosen AE, et al: Unipolar relatives in bipolar pedigrees: a search for elusive indicators of underlying bipolarity. Am J Med Genet 67:445–454, 1996

Bond TC, Rothschild AJ, Lerbinger J, et al: Delusional depression, family history, and DST response: a pilot study. Biol Psychiatry 21:1239–1246, 1986

Coryell W, Tsuang MT: Primary unipolar depression and the prognostic importance of delusions. Arch Gen Psychiatry 39:1181–1184, 1982

Coryell W, Pfohl B, Zimmerman M: The clinical and neuroendocrine features of psychotic depression. J Nerv Ment Dis 172:521–528, 1984

Craig SP, Buckle VJ, Lamouroux A, et al: Localization of the human dopamine beta hydroxylase (DBH) gene to chromosome 9q34. Cytogenet Cell Genet 48:48–50, 1988

Cubells JF, van Kammen DP, Kelley ME, et al: Dopamine beta-hydroxylase: two polymorphisms in linkage disequilibrium at the structural gene DBH associate with biochemical phenotypic variation. Hum Genet 102:533–540, 1998

Cubells JF, Price LH, Meyers BS, et al: Genotype-controlled analysis of plasma dopamine beta-hydroxylase activity in psychotic unipolar major depression. Biol Psychiatry 51:358–364, 2002

Detera-Wadleigh SD: Lithium-related genetics of bipolar disorder. Ann Med 33:272–285, 2001

Embi N, Rylatt DB, Cohen P: Glycogen synthase kinase-3 from rabbit skeletal muscle: separation from cyclic-AMP-dependent protein kinase and phosphorylase kinase. Eur J Biochem 107:519–527, 1980

Endicott J, Nee J, Coryell W, et al: Schizoaffective, psychotic and nonpsychotic depression: differential familial association. Compr Psychiatry 27:1–13, 1986

Frangos E, Athanassenas G, Tsitourides S, et al: Psychotic depressive disorder: a separate entity? J Affect Disord 5:259–265, 1983

Klein PS, Melton DA: A molecular mechanism for the effect of lithium on development. Proc Natl Acad Sci U S A 93:8455–8459, 1996

Leckman JF, Weisman MM, Prusoff BA, et al: Subtypes of depression: family study perspective. Arch Gen Psychiatry 41:833–838, 1984

Maj M, Starace F, Pirozzi R: A family study of DSM-III-R schizoaffective disorder, depressive subtype, compared with schizophrenia and psychotic and nonpsychotic major depression. Am J Psychiatry 148:612–616, 1991

Manji HK, Moore GJ, Chen G: Lithium up-regulates the cytoprotective protein Bcl-2 in the CNS in vivo: a role for neurotrophic and neuroprotective effects in manic depressive illness. J Clin Psychiatry 61:82–96, 2000

Meltzer HY, Cho HW, Carroll BJ, et al: Serum dopamine-beta-hydroxylase activity in the affective psychoses and schizophrenia: decreased activity in unipolar psychotically depressed patients. Arch Gen Psychiatry 33:585–591, 1976

Meyers BS, Alexopoulos GS, Kakuma T, et al: Decreased dopamine beta hydroxylase activity in unipolar geriatric delusional depression. Biol Psychiatry 45:448–452, 1999

Mod L, Rihmer Z, Magyar I, et al: Serum DBH activity in psychotic vs. nonpsychotic unipolar and bipolar depression. Psychiatry Res 19:331–333, 1986

Nelson WH, Khan A, Orr WW: Delusional depression: phenomenology, neuroendocrine function, and tricyclic antidepressant response. J Affect Disord 6:297–306, 1984

Price LH, Nelson JC, Charney DS, et al: Family history in delusional depression. J Affect Disord 6:109–114, 1984

Robertson D, Haile V, Perry SE, et al: Dopamine beta-hydroxylase deficiency: a genetic disorder of cardiovascular regulation. Hypertension 18:1–8, 1991

Salinas PC, Hall AC: Lithium and synaptic plasticity. Bipolar Disord 1:87–90, 1999

Sapru MK, Rao BS, Channabasavanna SM: Serum dopamine-beta-hydroxylase activity in clinical subtypes of depression. Acta Psychiatr Scand 80:474–478, 1989

Schatzberg AF, Rothschild AJ, Langlais PJ, et al: A corticosteroid/dopamine hypothesis for psychotic depression and related states. J Psychiatr Res 19:57–64, 1985

Serretti A, Macciardi F, Cusin C, et al: Dopamine receptor D4 gene is associated with delusional symptomatology in mood disorders. Psychiatry Res 80:129–136, 1998

Serretti A, Lattuada E, Catalano M, et al: Serotonin transporter gene not associated with psychotic symptomatology of mood disorders. Psychiatry Res 86:59–65, 1999a

Serretti A, Lilli R, Di Bella D, et al: Dopamine receptor D4 gene is not associated with major psychoses. Am J Med Genet 88:486–491, 1999b

Serretti A, Lilli R, Lorenzi C, et al: No association between serotonin-2A receptor gene polymorphism and psychotic symptomatology of mood disorders. Psychiatry Res 86:203–209, 1999c

Serretti A, Macciardi F, Catalano M, et al: Genetic variants of dopamine receptor D4 and psychopathology. Schizophr Bull 25:609–618, 1999d

Serretti A, Lilli R, Lorenzi C, et al: Serotonin-2C and serotonin-1A receptor genes are not associated with psychotic symptomatology of mood disorders. Am J Med Genet 96:161–166, 2000

Serretti A, Benedetti F, Mandelli L, et al: Association between GSK-3beta –50T/C polymorphism and personality and psychotic symptoms in mood disorders. Psychiatry Res 158:132–140, 2008

Stambolic V, Woodgett JR: Mitogen inactivation of glycogen synthase kinase-3 beta in intact cells via serine 9 phosphorylation. Biochem J 303:701–704, 1994

Wei J, Ramchand CN, Hemmings GP: Possible control of dopamine beta-hydroxylase via a codominant mechanism associated with the polymorphic (GT)n repeat at its gene locus in healthy individuals. Hum Genet 99:52–55, 1997

Wei J, Ramchand CN, Hemmings GP: TaqI polymorphic sites at the human dopamine beta-hydroxylase gene possibly associated with biochemical alterations of the catecholamine pathway in schizophrenia. Psychiatr Genet 8:19–24, 1998

Weissman MM, Prusoff BA, Merikangas KR: Is delusional depression related to bipolar disorder? Am J Psychiatry 141:892–893, 1984

Weissman MM, Warner V, Prusoff JK, et al: Delusional depression and bipolar spectrum: evidence for a possible association from a family study of children. Neuropsychopharmacology 1:257–264, 1988

Wilson AF, Elston RC, Siervogel RM, et al: Linkage of a gene regulating dopamine-beta-hydroxylase activity and the ABO blood group locus. Am J Hum Genet 42:160–166, 1988

Wood JG, Joyce PR, Miller AL, et al: A polymorphism in the dopamine beta-hydroxylase gene is associated with "paranoid ideation" in patients with major depression. Biol Psychiatry 51:365–376, 2002

Zabetian CP, Anderson GM, Buxbaum SG, et al: A quantitative-trait analysis of human plasma-dopamine beta-hydroxylase activity: evidence for a major functional polymorphism at the DBH locus. Am J Hum Genet 68:515–522, 2001

Recommended Reading

Cubells JF, Price LH, Meyers BS, et al: Genotype-controlled analysis of plasma dopamine beta-hydroxylase activity in psychotic unipolar major depression. Biol Psychiatry 51:358–364, 2002

Serretti A, Lattuada E, Catalano M, et al: Serotonin transporter gene not associated with psychotic symptomatology of mood disorders. Psychiatry Res 86:59–65, 1999

Weissman MM, Prusoff BA, Merikangas KR: Is delusional depression related to bipolar disorder? Am J Psychiatry 141:892–893, 1984

4

Biology

According to research results, the biology of psychotic depression differs from that of nonpsychotic depression. In this chapter, I review studies of the biology of psychotic depression, including those involving dysregulation of the hypothalamic-pituitary-adrenal (HPA) axis, the enzyme dopamine-β-hydroxylase, the dopaminergic system, the growth hormone (GH) response after administration of growth hormone–releasing hormone (GHRH), and the serotonergic system (see Table 4–1 for a summary of findings). I also discuss the use of neuroimaging, electroencephalographic measures, and P300 event-related potentials in studies of psychotic depression. Although many of the topics discussed in this chapter are in the realm of ongoing research, a few may be of current clinical utility (e.g., the dexamethasone suppression test [DST] in the differentiation of psychotic depression from schizophrenia [American Psychiatric Association 1987]).

Table 4–1. Biology of psychotic depression (relative to nonpsychotic depression)

↑	Hypothalamic-adrenal-pituitary axis dysregulation
↓	Dopamine-β-hydroxylase activity
?	Dopamine abnormality
?	Decreased growth hormone response to GHRH
?	Serotonin abnormality
↑	Ventricle-to-brain ratio
↓	REM latency
↓	REM activity

Note. GHRH = growth hormone–releasing hormone; REM = rapid eye movement.

Dysregulation of the Hypothalamic-Pituitary-Adrenal Axis

Patients with psychotic depression have marked dysregulation of the HPA axis, as exhibited by high rates of nonsuppression on the DST, with markedly elevated postdexamethasone cortisol levels, high levels of 24-hour urinary free cortisol (UFC), and an increased adrenocorticotropic hormone (ACTH) response to the dexamethasone/corticotropin-releasing hormone (DEX/CRH) test (see Table 4–2). The dysregulation of the HPA axis observed in psychotic depression is one of the most reliable biological alterations observed in psychiatric patients (American Psychiatric Association 1987; Rothschild 2003). Table 4–3 outlines HPA axis testing.

A meta-analysis of 12 different studies, with a combined sample size of approximately 1,000 depressed patients, indicated that when inpatient status was controlled for, increased rates of nonsuppression on the DST were associated with psychosis but not with melancholic symp-

Table 4–2. Hypothalamic-pituitary-adrenal axis abnormalities in psychotic depression (relative to nonpsychotic depression)

↑ Nonsuppression on dexamethasone suppression test
↑ 24-hour urinary free cortisol
↑ Adrenocorticotropic hormone response to dexamethasone/corticotropin-releasing hormone test

toms (Nelson and Davis 1997). The postdexamethasone cortisol nonsuppression rate was substantially higher in patients with psychotic depression (64%) than in nonpsychotic patients (41%) (Nelson and Davis 1997); however, the sensitivity and specificity were only 64% and 59%, respectively. Use of a postdexamethasone cortisol cutoff value higher than the traditional ≥5 µg/dL resulted in greater specificity for psychotic depression at the cost of sensitivity. One study found that 50% of the patients with psychotic depression had cortisol values ≥15 µg/dL, compared with only 7% of the patients with nonpsychotic depression (sensitivity of 50% and specificity of 93%), and that 43% of the patients with psychotic depression had cortisol values of ≥17 µg/dL, whereas none of the patients with nonpsychotic depression did (sensitivity of 43% and specificity of 100%) (Schatzberg et al. 1983). The DST may also discriminate well between patients with psychotic depression and patients with other psychoses, such as schizophrenia (American Psychiatric Association 1987). In one study, 57% of the patients with psychotic depression had postdexamethasone cortisol values greater than 14 µg/dL, whereas none of the patients with psychotic schizophrenia had values that high, and the mean postdexamethasone cortisol level for the patients with psychotic depression (13.0±8.1 µg/dL) was significantly higher than that for the patients with psychotic schizophrenia (2.4±2.8 µg/dL; $P<0.05$) (Rothschild et al. 1982).

Anton (1987) reported significant elevation in 24-hour measures of UFC levels in patients with psychotic depression. In this study, UFC, a

Table 4–3. Hypothalamic-pituitary-adrenal axis testing

Dexamethasone suppression test

Dexamethasone 1 mg at 2300 hours

Following day: Plasma cortisol drawn at 0800 hours and/or 1600 hours

24-hour urinary free cortisol

Person urinates in bottle for 24 hours

Dexamethasone/corticotropin-releasing hormone test

Dexamethasone 1.5 mg at 2300 hours

Following day:

1430 hours: Insertion of intravenous catheter

1500 hours: Measurement of plasma ACTH and cortisol

Injection of CRH 100 μg through intravenous catheter

Measurement of plasma ACTH and cortisol concentrations 30, 45, 60, and 75 minutes after CRH injection

Note. ACTH=adrenocorticotropic hormone; CRH=corticotropin-releasing hormone.

sensitive parameter of 24-hour cortisol production, was examined both before and after dexamethasone administration in 32 patients with major depression, 18 with psychotic features and 14 without psychotic features. Compared with patients without psychotic features, a significantly larger number of the patients with psychotic features had UFC excretion greater than 90 μg/24 hours before dexamethasone administration and greater than 20 μg/24 hours after dexamethasone administration. Although some clinical variables other than psychotic features differed between the two groups, these variables could not account for the UFC differences. The older patients (>55 years) in the psychotic depression group accounted for the high UFC excretion, suggesting an interaction between age and diagnosis (Anton 1987).

The combined DEX/CRH test more accurately assesses the activity of the HPA axis system (Holsboer et al. 1987; Holsboer-Trachsler et al. 1991) than does the DST (Heuser et al. 1994; Oshima et al. 2000), with greater sensitivity and specificity (Owashi et al. 2008). Owashi and colleagues (2008), who used the DEX/CRH test, described greater HPA activity in patients with psychotic depression than in patients with nonpsychotic depression. At admission, the psychotic depression group exhibited greater elevation of ACTH responses to the DEX/CRH test than did the nonpsychotic depression group. At discharge, the neuroendocrine responses to the DEX/CRH test of the psychotic depression group were still stronger than those of the nonpsychotic depression group, although the two groups had no significant differences in severity of depression. Significant longitudinal changes occurred in neuroendocrine responses to the DEX/CRH test between admission and discharge (Owashi et al. 2008).

The mechanism by which cortisol is associated with psychosis is not exactly clear, but both endogenous steroids (as in Cushing disease) and exogenous steroids have been associated with psychosis. Clearly, however, the greater HPA activity seen in patients with psychotic depression is not merely the result of greater severity of depression, the presence of endogenous features, or the psychosis per se, but rather is related to the interaction between the affective disorder and the psychosis. One group (Schatzberg and Rothschild 1988; Schatzberg et al. 1985) has hypothesized that the development of delusions in depressed patients is due to the effects of hypercortisolemia on dopaminergic systems, because glucocorticoids increase levels of dopamine in human plasma (Rothschild et al. 1984) and rat brain (Rothschild et al. 1985) and increase levels of homovanillic acid in rat brain (Wolkowitz et al. 1986) and human cerebrospinal fluid (CSF) (Banki et al. 1983). Another group (Duval et al. 2000) administered a central dopamine activity challenge, using apomorphine (a dopamine agonist that stimulates GH), and measured cortisol responses in healthy controls and patients with psychotic or nonpsychotic depression. Although the patients with psychotic depression showed increased activity of the HPA system (i.e., higher post-DST cortisol levels) compared with the patients with nonpsychotic depression or the healthy control subjects, the three groups had no differences in ACTH, cortisol, prolactin, or GH responses to apomorphine, suggesting a lack of a causal link between HPA axis hyperactivity and dopamine dysregulation (Duval et al. 2000). The same research group reported a blunted GH response to clonidine and concluded that this response implies the occurrence of a hyposensitivity of noradrenergic α_2 receptors in affective psychosis rather than dopamine system dysregulation (Mokrani et al. 2000). However, several older studies observed elevated levels of dopamine in plasma (Rothschild et al. 1987) or homovanillic acid (a dopamine metabolite) in either CSF or plasma of patients with psychotic depression (Schatzberg et al. 1995), and psychotic depression shows a strong clinical response to combined treatment with antidepressants and dopamine blockers (either typical or atypical antipsychotics) (see Chapter 6, "Treatment").

Rothschild and colleagues (1993) hypothesized that abnormal cortisol levels in patients with psychotic depression might also contribute to the profile of neuropsychological deficits observed. One study (Belanoff et al. 2001) found that patients with psychotic depression had both higher mean afternoon cortisol levels on the day of testing and more errors of commission (falsely believing they had been previously presented with words they had not seen) on the Wallach Memory Recognition Test compared with patients with nonpsychotic depression or psychiatrically healthy volunteers. This pattern is similar to that observed in healthy comparison subjects who were given corticosteroids (Belanoff 2001; Wolkowitz 1990).

Studies of the Dopaminergic System

Dopamine-β-Hydroxylase

A rather consistent neurochemical finding is reduced activity of dopamine-β-hydroxylase (DBH)—the enzyme that converts dopamine to norepinephrine—among patients with unipolar psychotic depression but not among those with bipolar psychotic depression (Schatzberg and Rothschild 1996). Five studies (Cubells et al. 2002; Meltzer et al. 1976; Meyers et al. 1999; Mod et al. 1986; Sapru et al. 1989)—but not a sixth (Lykouras et al. 1988)—showed that plasma DBH was significantly reduced in patients with psychotic depression compared with patients with nonpsychotic depression or psychiatrically healthy controls. Lykouras et al. observed no significant differences in DBH activity between patients with psychotic depression and patients with nonpsychotic depression. A seventh small study showed reductions in DBH that did not reach statistical significance (Eisemann et al. 1983). Because serum DBH did not increase for most patients immediately following successful treatment, Meltzer and colleagues (1976) suggested that DBH may be a trait-dependent rather than a state-dependent finding in patients with psychotic depression. Low CSF DBH activity has also been associated with psychosis induced by disulfiram (Major et al. 1979) and cocaine (Cubells et al. 2000). However, one study (Hamner and Gold 1998), but not another (Meltzer et al. 1976), observed elevated rather than reduced DBH activity in psychotic patients with bipolar disorder compared with psychiatrically healthy controls, and higher DBH levels in patients with schizophrenia than in patients with psychotic depression (Meltzer et al. 1976). These authors suggest that low DBH may be a trait-specific rather than a state-specific vulnerability factor. Schatzberg and colleagues (1985) hypothesized that the low levels of DBH activity in psychotic depression might be a potential marker of relative risk for developing pronounced increases in dopamine levels in the face of chronic elevation of cortisol levels.

Dopamine and Homovanillic Acid

Several studies have demonstrated that based on measurements of dopamine or its metabolite homovanillic acid (HVA), patients with psychotic depression exhibit an activation of the dopaminergic system that is not seen in patients with nonpsychotic depression. Patients with psychotic depression demonstrate significantly higher levels of unconjugated plasma dopamine both before and after administration of dexamethasone (Rothschild et al. 1987). Aberg-Wistedt and colleagues (1985) reported that patients with psychotic depression had significantly higher concentrations of HVA in CSF than did patients with nonpsychotic depression. Studies of plasma HVA also indicate that patients with psychotic depression have greater activation of dopaminergic systems than do patients with nonpsychotic depression. Mazure and colleagues (1987) reported that plasma HVA levels were significantly higher in patients with psychotic depression than in melancholic patients with nonpsychotic depression, who in turn had higher levels than nonmelancholic patients with nonpsychotic depression. This report is consistent with the earlier observation of Devanand and colleagues (1985), who reported that plasma HVA levels were significantly higher in women with psychotic depression than in women with nonpsychotic depression. A trend toward relative blunting of the plasma HVA response to dexamethasone in patients with psychotic depression compared with patients with nonpsychotic depression has also been described (Wolkowitz et al. 1985, 1989).

Growth Hormone Response to Growth Hormone–Releasing Hormone

In a study of the GH response after administration of GHRH in patients with psychotic depression, Owashi and colleagues (2008) observed significant differences between psychotic and nonpsychotic depressed patients, although not all studies are in agreement (Contreras et al. 2007; Duval et al. 2000). Evaluation of the hypothalamic-pituitary-somatotropic axis is another way of assessing dopaminergic function, because several interactions between GHRH and dopaminergic function have been reported (see Crespi et al. 1985; Vance et al. 1987). Dopamine receptor agonists such as apomorphine stimulate GH secretion, and decreased (Pitchot et al. 1990–1991) or unchanged (Lal

1988) GH responses to apomorphine have been reported in patients with depression. The blunted GH responses to apomorphine might be the result of depression-related alteration at the hypothalamic-pituitary level.

In the GHRH test, the patient fasts (except water and prescribed drugs) beginning at 2130 hours the previous night. On the day of examination, an intravenous catheter with heparinized physiological saline is inserted into a forearm vein at 0830 hours, and human GHRH 100 mg is injected intravenously at 0900 hours, immediately after the first blood collection. Serum GH concentrations are then measured 15, 30, 60, and 90 minutes postinjection (Owashi et al. 2008).

Owashi and colleagues (2008) observed that at admission to an inpatient unit, patients with psychotic depression exhibited a tendency toward decreased GH responses to GHRH compared with patients with nonpsychotic depression. By the time of discharge, all psychotic features had improved and significant longitudinal change had occurred in the GHRH test results in the psychotic depression group, and no differences in GHRH test results existed between psychotic and nonpsychotic depressed patients. These observations suggest that dysregulation of GH function may be related to psychotic features in depression and that GH function is state dependent in being specifically associated with psychotic features. These findings are in contrast to those of two other studies (Contreras et al. 2007; Duval et al. 2000). Duval and colleagues (2000) reported no significant differences in GH responses to apomorphine (a dopamine agonist that stimulates GH) in patients with psychotic depression versus patients with nonpsychotic depression, although Owashi and colleagues (2008) criticized the study for not including body mass index as a covariate in the analysis. When Owashi and colleagues did not include body mass index as a covariate in their own analysis, they observed no significant differences or even a tendency toward significant differences in GH responses at admission between patients with psychotic depression and patients with nonpsychotic depression. In the second study, Contreras and colleagues (2007) observed no significant differences in GH responses to the GHRH test in patients with psychotic versus nonpsychotic melancholic depression.

Studies of the Serotonergic System

A number of studies have addressed serotonin (5-HT) activity in patients with psychotic depression. Healy and colleagues (1986) reported that 5-HT uptake into platelets was significantly higher in patients with psychotic depression than in patients with nonpsychotic depression. In that study, endogenously depressed patients demonstrated a relative decrease in uptake in comparison with controls, but psychotically depressed patients did not. After clinical recovery, psychotic depressed and nonpsychotic depressed patients showed no differences in 5-HT uptake into platelets, suggesting that increased 5-HT uptake in psychotic depression reflects a state- rather than a trait-dependent marker.

Aberg-Wistedt and colleagues (1985) reported that CSF levels of both HVA and 5-hydroxyindoleacetic acid (5-HIAA) were significantly higher in patients with psychotic depression than in patients with nonpsychotic depression (see subsection "Dopamine and Homovanillic Acid"). In that study, as well as others using a variety of patient groups and controls, HVA and 5-HIAA levels significantly and positively correlated with each other. Both Aberg-Wistedt and colleagues (1985) and Agren and Terenius (1985) reported that the ratio of HVA to 5-HIAA appeared either to separate patients with psychotic depression from patients with nonpsychotic depression or to correlate more robustly with psychotic symptoms. These findings suggest that HVA and dopamine may be more closely related to psychotic features in depression than is 5-HT or 5-HIAA. Still, the observations that 5-HT metabolite levels are higher in patients with psychotic depression do suggest a possible role for 5-HT. Two studies found no differences in 5-HIAA levels in patients with psychotic depression and patients with nonpsychotic depression. In one study measuring CSF levels, only a small number of subjects were assessed (Sweeney et al. 1978), and in the other, urinary

5-HIAA levels were not higher in the patients with psychotic depression (Lykouras et al. 1988); however, the patients were not required to be drug free for inclusion in the Lykouras et al. study. Furthermore, because urinary 5-HIAA is heavily influenced by diet, its validity as a marker of central 5-HT activity is questionable.

Clinical responses observed with amoxapine (which has both 5-HT agonist and dopamine antagonist effects) (Anton and Sexauer 1983) have hinted at the possibility that serotonin type-2 (5-HT_2) receptors may be involved in psychotic depression, but their purported role has not been supported by genetic studies (see Chapter 3, "Family Studies and Genetics"). A few studies have also found lower levels of CSF 5-HIAA (Mendels et al. 1972) or urinary MHPG (3-methoxy-4-hydroxyphenylglycol) (Sweeney et al. 1978) in patients with psychotic depression than in patients with nonpsychotic depression. One study examined the relationship between exogenous 5-HT (a 5-HT precursor) and serum cortisol and found that patients with psychotic depression had less of a 5-HT–induced increase in cortisol compared with patients with nonpsychotic depression, but it is unclear whether this finding may have been due to higher cortisol at baseline (Meltzer et al. 1984).

Neuroimaging Studies

Multiple groups have reported enlarged cerebral ventricles in patients with psychotic depression (Jones et al. 1994; Luchins and Meltzer 1983; Rothschild et al. 1989; Schlegel and Kretzschmar 1987; Targum et al. 1983). The first study to observe enlarged ventricles in melancholic patients with psychotic depression failed to find statistically significant differences overall, but one-fourth of the psychotic depression sample, compared with none of the nonpsychotic depression sample, had a mean ventricle-to-brain ratio (VBR) that was at least two standard deviations larger than that of the control group (Targum et al. 1983). Luchins and Meltzer (1983) found the mean VBR to be 44% larger in patients with bipolar or unipolar psychotic depression than in a slightly younger sample with nonpsychotic depression. Fifty-six percent (5/9) of the patients with psychotic depression but only 11% (1/9) of the patients with nonpsychotic depression had VBRs greater than one standard deviation larger than the control group's mean VBR. The authors contrasted their findings to reports at the time that the VBR was smaller in patients with schizophrenia. In a larger study, Schlegel and Kretzschmar (1987) found increased VBRs in patients with psychotic affective illness, as well as in older patients and male patients, but did not find an association between VBR and DST results or between unipolar patients and bipolar patients.

In a group including bipolar patients, Rothschild and colleagues (1989) found that differences in VBR were more pronounced in patients with psychotic depression than in patients with nonpsychotic depression. One hundred percent of the patients with psychotic depression had a cella media VBR of at least 0.61, compared with 58% of nonpsychotic depressed patients (P=0.03). Similar proportions were observed for DST nonsuppressors versus suppressors, although these results did not reach statistical significance (P=0.067). Sulcal size, a possible indicator of "atrophy," was also judged to be larger in the left and right inferior parietal areas (Brodmann areas 39 and 40) of patients with psychotic depression (Rothschild et al. 1989).

In a study of 54 patients with affective psychosis, Jones and colleagues (1994) similarly found larger third ventricles among patients with psychotic affective illness but observed that no clear threshold existed between "normal" and "enlarged" ventricles. O'Brien and colleagues (1997), in a study of older patients, found no differences in abnormalities in temporal lobe atrophy, periventricular white matter lesions, DST results, or cognitive testing results between the psychotic depression sample and the nonpsychotic depression sample. They did find a greater number of vascular risk factors and a nonsignificant trend toward a greater number of deep white matter lesions in the psychotic depression sample. Kim and colleagues (1999), in their study of depressed patients age 55 years or older, found that the absolute volume of prefrontal cortex was smaller in the group with psychotic depression compared with the group with nonpsychotic depression, and that this decreased volume correlated with performance on the Wisconsin Card Sorting Test.

Finally, in a recent magnetic resonance imaging study by Keller et al. (2008), patients with psychotic depression had significantly smaller mean amygdala volume relative to depressed patients without psychosis and healthy comparison subjects. However, contrary to the conclusions of previous meta-analyses (Videbach and Raunkilde 2004; Campbell and MacQueen 2006), Keller et al. did not find left or right hippocampal volume differences in patients with psychotic or nonpsychotic depression relative to healthy comparison subjects.

Electroencephalographic Studies

Electroencephalographic studies of psychotic depression are uncommon. In an electroencephalographic sleep study, Thase and colleagues (1986) found that patients with psychotic depression exhibited increased wakefulness, decreased rapid eye movement (REM) sleep, and decreased REM activity compared with patients with nonpsychotic depression, after age, severity, and agitation were controlled. REM latency also appeared to be a marker for duration of illness; patients with recent-onset psychotic depression had marked initial insomnia and long REM latency, whereas patients with illnesses of longer duration had extremely short REM latencies (Thase et al. 1986).

Another study reported abnormal electroencephalographic findings in 17% of a medicated sample of patients with mood-incongruent psychotic depression and 10% of patients with mood-congruent psychotic depression, compared with 3.2% of healthy control subjects (Inui et al. 1998). Furthermore, 33% of the patients with mood-incongruent psychotic depression were found to have epileptiform electroencephalographic variants, compared with 0% of the patients with mood-congruent psychotic depression. Inui and colleagues argued for a possible similar biological substrate for "atypical psychoses" (mood-incongruent psychotic depression, schizoaffective disorder, and schizophreniform disorder, all of which had similar proportions of epileptiform variants). However, findings from outcome studies have indicated that mood-incongruent psychotic depression has outcomes much more similar to those of mood-congruent psychotic depression than to outcomes of schizoaffective disorder or schizophrenia (Coryell et al. 1982).

P300 Studies

Decreased amplitude and increased latency in P300 event-related potentials have been reported in patients with schizophrenia, but few studies have been done using P300 in patients with psychotic depression. Melancholic patients with psychotic depression were found to have decreased P300 amplitude compared with melancholic patients with nonpsychotic depression (Santosh et al. 1994). In a study of 22 unipolar depressed patients (82% with major depression, 18% with dysthymia), Kaustio and colleagues (2002) found that scores on the Psychoticism subscale of the Symptom Checklist–90, a 90-item symptom checklist, correlated with an overall reduction in P300 amplitude, especially over the left temporocentral electrode chain. However, the sample was selected for depression rather than psychosis, and none of these subjects had particularly high Psychoticism scores. In contrast, Salisbury and colleagues (1998) observed no differences in left temporal amplitude between patients with affective psychosis and healthy controls, but only 14% of those with psychosis had unipolar major depression.

Key Clinical Points

- Patients with psychotic depression are biologically distinct from patients with nonpsychotic depression.
- Patients with psychotic depression exhibit marked dysregulation of the hypothalamic-pituitary-adrenal axis (HPA) compared with patients with nonpsychotic depression.

- Patients with psychotic depression exhibit lower levels of dopamine-β-hydroxylase (DBH) activity compared with patients with nonpsychotic depression.
- Neuroimaging studies have found larger ventricle-to-brain ratios and smaller amygdala volumes in patients with psychotic depression compared with patients with nonpsychotic depression.
- Measures of HPA axis activity (e.g., the dexamethasone suppression test) and sleep studies may be clinically useful in differentiating schizophrenia spectrum disorders from psychotic depression, because these two disorders differ significantly in HPA axis activity and electroencephalographic measures.

References

Aberg-Wistedt A, Wistedt B, Bertilsson L: Higher CSF levels of HVA and 5-HIAA in delusional compared to nondelusional depression (letter). Arch Gen Psychiatry 42:925–926, 1985

Agren H, Terenius L: Hallucinations in patients with major depression: interactions between CSF monoaminergic and endorphinergic indices. J Affect Disord 9:25–34, 1985

American Psychiatric Association: The dexamethasone suppression test: an overview of its current status in psychiatry. The APA Task Force on Laboratory Tests in Psychiatry. Am J Psychiatry 144:1253–1262, 1987

Anton RF: Urinary free cortisol in psychotic depression. Biol Psychiatry 22:24–34, 1987

Anton RF, Sexauer JD: Efficacy of amoxapine in psychotic depression. Am J Psychiatry 140:1344–1347, 1983

Banki CM, Arató M, Papp Z: Cerebrospinal fluid biochemical examinations: do they reflect clinical or biological differences? Biol Psychiatry 18:1033–1044, 1983

Belanoff JK, Kalehzan M, Sund B, et al: Cortisol activity and cognitive changes in psychotic major depression. Am J Psychiatry 158:1612–1616, 2001

Campbell S, MacQueen G: An update on regional brain volume differences associated with mood disorders. Curr Opin Psychiatry 19:25–33, 2006

Contreras F, Menchon JM, Urretavizcaya M, et al: Hormonal differences between psychotic and non-psychotic melancholic depression. J Affect Disord 100:65–73, 2007

Coryell W, Tsuang MT, McDaniel J: Psychotic features in major depression: is mood congruence important? J Affect Disord 4:227–236, 1982

Crespi F, Paret J, Keane PE, et al: Growth hormone–releasing factor modifies dopaminergic but not serotonergic activity in the arcuate nucleus of hypothalamus in the rat, as recorded in vivo by differential pulse voltammetry. Brain Res 348:367–370, 1985

Cubells JF, Kranzler HR, McCance-Katz E, et al: A haplotype at the DBH locus, associated with low plasma dopamine beta-hydroxylase activity, also associates with cocaine-induced paranoia. Mol Psychiatry 5:56–63, 2000

Cubells JF, Price LH, Meyers BS, et al: Genotype-controlled analysis of plasma dopamine beta-hydroxylase activity in psychotic unipolar major depression. Biol Psychiatry 51:358–364, 2002

Devanand DP, Bowers MB, Hoffman FJ, et al: Elevated plasma homovanillic acid in depressed females with melancholia and psychosis. Psychiatry Res 15:1–4, 1985

Duval F, Mokrani MC, Crocq MA, et al: Dopaminergic function and the cortisol response to dexamethasone in psychotic depression. Prog Neuropsychopharmacol Biol Psychiatry 24:207–225, 2000

Eisemann M, Ericsson U, Von Knorring L, et al: Serum dopamine-beta-hydroxylase in diagnostic subgroups of depressed patients and in relation to their personality characteristics. Neuropsychobiology 9:193–196, 1983

Hamner MB, Gold PB: Plasma dopamine beta-hydroxylase activity in psychotic and non-psychotic post-traumatic stress disorder. Psychiatry Res 77:175–181, 1998

Healy D, O'Halloran A, Carney PA, et al: Platelet 5-HT uptake in delusional and nondelusional depressions. J Affect Disord 10:233–239, 1986

Heuser I, Yassouridis A, Holsboer F: The combined dexamethasone/CRH test: a refined laboratory test for psychiatric disorders. J Psychiatr Res 28:341–356, 1994

Holsboer F, von Bardeleben U, Wiedemann K, et al: Serial assessment of corticotropin-releasing hormone response after dexamethasone in depression: implications for pathophysiology of DST nonsuppression. Biol Psychiatry 22:228–234, 1987

Holsboer-Trachsler E, Stohler R, Hatzinger M: Repeated administration of the combined dexamethasone–human corticotropin releasing hormone stimulation test during treatment of depression. Psychiatry Res 38:163–171, 1991

Inui K, Motomura E, Okushima R, et al: Electroencephalographic findings in patients with DSM-IV mood disorder, schizophrenia, and other psychotic disorders. Biol Psychiatry 43:69–75, 1998

Jones PB, Harvey I, Lewis SW, et al: Cerebral ventricle dimensions as risk factors for schizophrenia and affective psychosis: an epidemiological approach to analysis. Psychol Med 24:995–1011, 1994

Kaustio O, Partanen J, Valkonen-Korhonen M, et al: Affective and psychotic symptoms relate to different types of P300 alteration in depressive disorder. J Affect Disord 71:43–50, 2002

Keller J, Shen L, Gomez RG, et al: Hippocampal and amygdalar volumes in psychotic and nonpsychotic unipolar depression. Am J Psychiatry 165:872–880, 2008

Kim DK, Kim BL, Sohn SE, et al: Candidate neuroanatomic substrates of psychosis in old-aged depression. Prog Neuropsychopharmacol Biol Psychiatry 23:793–807, 1999

Lal S: Apomorphine in the evaluation of dopaminergic function in man. Prog Neuropsychopharmacol Biol Psychiatry 12:117–164, 1988

Luchins DJ, Meltzer HY: Ventricular size and psychosis in affective disorder. Biol Psychiatry 18:1197–1198, 1983

Lykouras E, Markianos M, Malliaras D, et al: Neurochemical variables in delusional depression. Am J Psychiatry 145:214–217, 1988

Major LF, Lerner P, Ballenger JC, et al: Dopamine-beta-hydroxylase in the cerebrospinal fluid: relationship to disulfiram-induced psychosis. Biol Psychiatry 14:337–344, 1979

Mazure CM, Bowers MB, Hoffman F, et al: Plasma catecholamine metabolites in subtypes of major depression. Biol Psychiatry 22:1469–1472, 1987

Meltzer HY, Cho HW, Carroll BJ, et al: Serum dopamine-beta-hydroxylase activity in the affective psychoses and schizophrenia: decreased activity in unipolar psychotically depressed patients. Arch Gen Psychiatry 33:585–591, 1976

Meltzer HY, Perline R, Tricou BJ, et al: Effect of 5-hydroxytryptophan on serum cortisol levels in major affective disorders, II: relation to suicide, psychosis, and depressive symptoms. Arch Gen Psychiatry 41:379–387, 1984

Mendels J, Frazer A, Fitzgerald RG, et al: Biogenic amine metabolites in cerebrospinal fluid of depressed and manic patients. Science 175:1380–1382, 1972

Meyers BS, Alexopoulos GS, Kakuma T, et al: Decreased dopamine beta-hydroxylase activity in unipolar geriatric delusional depression. Biol Psychiatry 45:448–452, 1999

Mod L, Rihmer Z, Magyar I, et al: Serum DBH activity in psychotic vs. non-psychotic unipolar and bipolar depression. Psychiatry Res 19:331–333, 1986

Mokrani MC, Duval F, Diep TS, et al: Multihormonal responses to clonidine in patients with affective and psychotic symptoms. Psychoneuroendocrinology 25:741–752, 2000

Nelson JC, Davis JM: DST studies in psychotic depression: a meta-analysis. Am J Psychiatry 154:1497–1503, 1997

O'Brien JT, Ames D, Schweitzer I, et al: Clinical, magnetic resonance imaging and endocrinological differences between delusional and non-delusional depression in the elderly. Int J Geriatr Psychiatry 12:211–218, 1997

Oshima A, Yamashita S, Owashi T, et al: The differential ACTH responses to combined dexamethasone/CRH administration in major depressive and dysthymic disorders. J Psychiatr Res 34:325–328, 2000

Owashi T, Otsubo T, Oshima A, et al: Longitudinal neuroendocrine changes assessed by dexamethasone/CRH and growth hormone releasing hormone tests in psychotic depression. Psychoneuroendocrinology 33:152–161, 2008

Pitchot W, Hansenne M, Moreno AG, et al: Psychopathological correlates of dopaminergic disturbances in major depression. Neuropsychobiology 24:169–172, 1990–1991

Rothschild AJ: The hypothalamic-pituitary-adrenal axis and psychiatric illness, in Psychoneuroendocrinology. Edited by Wolkowitz OM, Rothschild AJ. Washington, DC, American Psychiatric Publishing, 2003, pp 139–163

Rothschild AJ, Schatzberg AF, Rosenbaum AH, et al: The dexamethasone suppression test as a discriminator among subtypes of psychotic patients. Br J Psychiatry 141:471–474, 1982

Rothschild AJ, Langlais PJ, Schatzberg AF, et al: Dexamethasone increases plasma free dopamine in man. J Psychiatr Res 18:217–223, 1984

Rothschild AJ, Langlais PJ, Schatzberg AF, et al: The effects of a single acute dose of dexamethasone on monoamine and metabolite levels in rat brain. Life Sci 36:2491–2501, 1985

Rothschild AJ, Schatzberg AF, Langlais PJ, et al: Psychotic and non-psychotic depressions, I: comparison of plasma catecholamines and cortisol measures. Psychiatry Res 20:143–153, 1987

Rothschild AJ, Benes F, Hebben N, et al: Relationships between brain CT scan findings and cortisol in psychotic and non-psychotic depressed patients. Biol Psychiatry 26:565–575, 1989

Rothschild AJ, Samson JA, Bond TC, et al: Hypothalamic-pituitary-adrenal axis activity and one-year outcome in depression. Biol Psychiatry 34:392–400, 1993

Salisbury DF, Shenton ME, Sherwood AR, et al: First-episode schizophrenic psychosis differs from first-episode affective psychosis and controls in P300 amplitude over left temporal lobe. Arch Gen Psychiatry 55:173–180, 1998

Santosh PJ, Malhotra S, Raghunathan M, et al: A study of P300 in melancholic depression: correlation with psychotic features. Biol Psychiatry 35:474–479, 1994

Sapru MK, Rao BS, Channabasavanna SM: Serum dopamine-beta-hydroxylase activity in clinical subtypes of depression. Acta Psychiatr Scand 80:474–478, 1989

Schatzberg AF, Rothschild AJ: The roles of glucocorticoid and dopaminergic systems in delusional (psychotic) depression. Ann N Y Acad Sci 537:462–471, 1988

Schatzberg AF, Rothschild AJ: Psychotic (delusional) major depression: should it be included as a distinct syndrome in DSM-IV? in DSM-IV Sourcebook, Vol 2. Edited by Widiger TA, Frances AJ, Pincus HA, et al. Washington, DC, American Psychiatric Press, 1996, pp 127–180

Schatzberg AF, Rothschild AJ, Stahl JB, et al: The dexamethasone suppression test: identification of subtypes of depression. Am J Psychiatry 140:88–91, 1983

Schatzberg AF, Rothschild AJ, Langlais PJ, et al: A corticosteroid/dopamine hypothesis for psychotic depression and related states. J Psychiatr Res 19:57–64, 1985

Schatzberg AF, Posener JA, Rothschild A: The role of dopamine in psychotic depression. Clin Neuropharmacol 18 (suppl 1):S1–S8, 1995

Schlegel S, Kretzschmar K: Computed tomography in affective disorders, part I: ventricular and sulcal measurements. Biol Psychiatry 22:4–14, 1987

Sweeney D, Nelson C, Bowers M, et al: Delusional versus nondelusional depression: neurochemical differences. Lancet 2:100–101, 1978

Targum SD, Rosen LN, DeLisi LE, et al: Cerebral ventricular size in major depressive disorder: association with delusional symptoms. Biol Psychiatry 18:329–336, 1983

Thase ME, Kupfer DJ, Ulrich RF: Electroencephalographic sleep in psychotic depression: a valid subtype? Arch Gen Psychiatry 43:886–893, 1986

Vance ML, Kaiser DL, Frohman LA, et al: Role of dopamine in the regulation of growth hormone secretion: dopamine and bromocriptine augment growth hormone (GH)-releasing hormone-stimulated GH secretion in normal man. J Clin Endocrinol Metab 64:1136–1141, 1987

Videbach P, Raunkilde B: Hippocampal volume and depression: a meta-analysis of MRI studies. Am J Psychiatry 161:1957–1966, 2004

Wolkowitz OM, Sutton ME, Doran AR, et al: Dexamethasone increases plasma HVA but not MHPG in normal humans. Psychiatry Res 16:101–109, 1985

Wolkowitz OM, Sutton M, Loula M, et al: Chronic corticosterone administration in rats: behavioral and biochemical evidence of increased central dopaminergic activity. Eur J Pharmacol 122:329–338, 1986

Wolkowitz OM, Doran A, Breier A, et al: Specificity of HVA response to dexamethasone in psychotic depression. Psychiatry Res 29:177–186, 1989

Wolkowitz OM, Reus VI, Weingartner H, et al: Cognitive effects of corticosteroids. Am J Psychiatry 147:1297–1303, 1990

Recommended Reading

Nelson JC, Davis JM: DST studies in psychotic depression: a meta-analysis. Am J Psychiatry 154:1497–1503, 1997

Rothschild AJ: The hypothalamic-pituitary-adrenal axis and psychiatric illness, in Psychoneuroendocrinology. Edited by Wolkowitz OM, Rothschild AJ. Washington, DC, American Psychiatric Publishing, 2003, pp 139–163

Schatzberg AF, Rothschild AJ: Psychotic (delusional) major depression: should it be included as a distinct syndrome in DSM-IV? in DSM-IV Sourcebook, Vol. 2. Edited by Widiger TA, Frances AJ, Pincus HA, et al. Washington, DC, American Psychiatric Press, 1996, pp 127–180

5

Diagnosis and Assessment

Clinical Presentation

Psychotic depression is often not diagnosed accurately because the psychosis may be subtle, intermittent, or concealed, leading to a misdiagnosis of nonpsychotic depression (Rothschild and Schatzberg 1993). However, a correct diagnosis is necessary before a patient with psychotic depression can be treated effectively. Improper diagnosis of psychotic depression as another psychotic disorder such as schizophrenia or failure to recognize the psychotic features during a major depressive episode will defer the use of effective treatment modalities. Recent data from the National Institute of Mental Health (NIMH) Study of the Pharmacotherapy of Psychotic Depression (STOP-PD) (Andreescu et al. 2007) suggest that suboptimal treatment of psychotic depression may be occurring at an alarming rate. Delaying the start of effective therapeutics may increase morbidity and mortality, as well as health care costs.

Assessment

For any psychiatric disorder, a medical workup should be done to rule out possible organic causes of the patient's symptoms. This assessment is particularly important for a patient experiencing a first episode of psychotic depression. As outlined in Table 5–1, the initial evaluation requires a thorough history, a physical examination, and laboratory investigations to exclude an organic cause. Important tests include a complete blood count; measures of electrolytes, blood urea nitrogen, creatinine, glucose, vitamin B_{12}, folate, and calcium; thyroid function tests; urinalysis; urine culture if the patient has fever; and a urine drug screen. A careful neurological assessment is essential; this includes a computed tomographic or magnetic resonance imaging scan of the head to rule out the presence of a brain tumor or a stroke related to ischemia (vascular occlusion) or hemorrhage (uncontrolled hypertension, ruptured arteriovenous malformation, or aneurysm).

According to DSM-IV-TR criteria (American Psychiatric Association 2000), the diagnosis of psychotic depression cannot be made unless the patient experiences delusions or hallucinations in the context of a major depressive episode (see Chapter 1, "Introduction"). The psychotic features can be classified as either mood-congruent or mood-incongruent psychotic features (see Table 5–2).

The detection of delusions and hallucinations is often difficult in patients with psychotic depression because these individuals are frequently paranoid and suspicious and can be concerned that others will think they are "crazy" (Rothschild and Schatzberg 1993); consequently, they tend to keep their psychotic thoughts to themselves. Therefore, it is not merely an academic exercise to consider what else, besides the delusions and hallucinations, differs between patients with psychotic depression and patients with nonpsychotic depression. In fact, a number of research groups have explored whether other characteristics may help in distinguishing patients with psychotic depression from those with nonpsychotic depression (see Table 5–3).

Table 5–1. Initial evaluation of a patient with a first episode of psychotic depression

History	Thyroid function tests
Physical examination	Calcium
Complete blood count	Urinalysis
Electrolytes	Urine culture (if fever present)
Blood urea nitrogen	Urine drug screen
Creatinine	Neurological assessment
Glucose	CT or MRI of brain
Vitamin B_{12}	
Folate	

Note. CT = computed tomography; MRI = magnetic resonance imaging.

Several groups have reported that patients with psychotic depression demonstrate a more frequent and severe psychomotor disturbance (either retardation or agitation) than do patients with nonpsychotic depression (Charney and Nelson 1981; Coryell et al. 1984; Frances et al. 1981; Glassman and Roose 1981; Lykouras et al. 1986; J.C. Nelson and Bowers 1978). When compared with patients with nonpsychotic depression, patients with psychotic depression have also been reported to exhibit more pronounced paranoid symptoms (Frances et al. 1981; Lykouras et al. 1986), cognitive impairment (Basso and Bornstein 1999; Belanoff et al. 2001; Jeste et al. 1996; E.B. Nelson et al. 1998; Rothschild et al. 1989; Schatzberg et al. 2000; Simpson et al. 1999), hopelessness (Frances et al. 1981), hypochondriasis (Coryell et al. 1984; Glassman and Roose 1981), anxiety (Charney and Nelson 1981; Glassman and Roose 1981), early insomnia (Frances et al. 1981; Lykouras et al. 1986), middle insomnia (Lykouras et al. 1986), and constipation (Parker et al. 1991). Also, unlike endogenously depressed nonpsychotic patients, patients with psychotic depression do not show a diurnal vari-

Table 5–2. Mood-congruent and mood-incongruent psychotic features in psychotic depression

Mood-congruent psychotic features: Delusions or hallucinations whose content is entirely consistent with the typical depressive themes of personal inadequacy, guilt, disease, death, nihilism, or deserved punishment.

Mood-incongruent psychotic features: Delusions or hallucinations whose content does not involve typical depressive themes of personal inadequacy, guilt, disease, death, nihilism, or deserved punishment. Included are such symptoms as persecutory delusions (not directly related to depressive themes), thought insertion, thought broadcasting, and delusions of control.

Source. American Psychiatric Association 2000.

ation in mood (Parker et al. 1991). Finally, in a recent study of 1,112 outpatients with major depression, the presence of a psychomotor disturbance, insomnia, indecisiveness, and suicidal ideation was predictive of psychotic depression (as opposed to nonpsychotic depression), even after the effects of demographic characteristics and other symptoms were controlled (Gaudiano et al. 2008).

Differential Diagnosis and Common Misdiagnoses

Psychotic Versus Nonpsychotic Depression

Because patients with psychotic depression are often guarded regarding their psychotic thinking, clinicians have difficulty correctly diagnosing psychotic or nonpsychotic depression. Many patients have told me (once they were better) that they feared that if they confided their thoughts to family, friends, or clinicians, they would be thought of as "crazy," and, therefore, the patients frequently kept their psychotic thinking to themselves. A further challenge in making an accurate di-

Table 5–3. Signs and symptoms of psychotic depression (relative to nonpsychotic depression)

Delusions and hallucinations	Increased somatic complaints
Increased guilt	Increased paranoia
Increased psychomotor disturbance (either retardation or agitation)	Increased hopelessness
	Increased hypochondriasis
Absent diurnal variation	Increased anxiety
Greater cognitive impairment	Increased early and middle insomnia

agnosis is that the delusions in psychotic depression often have an air of plausibility to them (e.g., "I'm dying from cancer," "I lost my company millions of dollars," "I've committed a crime"). In many cases, the clinician may not miss the symptom (e.g., guilt, poverty, persecution) but may not recognize that the symptom is a delusion. In particular, distinguishing between delusional guilt and nondelusional guilt can be difficult. Guilt is a common symptom of depression, and although a patient's guilt may be beyond what is typically expected in depression, the point at which guilt becomes delusional is often not clear. Consequently, although the symptoms of major depression are readily apparent to the clinician, the psychosis may be missed, which can lead to poor treatment (see Chapter 6, "Treatment"), underappreciation of the risk of suicide (see Chapter 10, "Special Populations and Issues"), and a lack of awareness of the amount of time needed for recovery.

Recent data from the National Institute of Mental Health STOP-PD (Rothschild et al. 2008) indicate that clinicians indeed frequently miss the diagnosis of psychotic depression, in large part because they do not recognize the psychotic features. In 27% of a possible 130 correct diagnoses in a well-characterized sample of patients with a research diagnosis of psychotic depression, a diagnosis of psychotic depression was not considered. The rate of missed diagnoses in this study is likely a conservative estimate of the rate in the general clinical population, because the study excluded patients with comorbid conditions, such as a history of substance abuse in the past 3 months, or unstable medical conditions. Psychotic depression was most commonly misdiagnosed as major depressive disorder without psychotic features, depression not otherwise specified, or mood disorder not otherwise specified. Strikingly, no patients with missed diagnoses were considered to have a psychotic disorder. This finding suggests that the physicians were missing the psychosis rather than the mood disorder.

Psychotic Depression Suspected but No Delusional Symptoms Elicited

When I suspect that a depressed patient may have psychotic symptoms but the patient is not disclosing them in an interview, I frequently use one of two strategies. The first is to ask the patient's permission to speak with a family member or to invite a family member to come with the patient to the next appointment. The following is an exchange that occurred when a family member attended an appointment with a patient:

> **Dr. Rothschild:** Have you had any unusual thoughts?
> **Patient:** No.
> **Dr. Rothschild:** Do you have feelings of paranoia?
> **Patient:** No.
> **Family member:** Tell Dr. Rothschild about the car across the street.
> **Patient:** Oh, that.

The patient then described a parked car that he believed contained FBI agents who were on a stakeout and were following him everywhere he went. The family member prompted the patient to explain a rather detailed delusional system; however, the patient previously had answered in the negative to my questions regarding paranoia and unusual thoughts because, to him, the delusional system was "real" and was not an example of unusual thoughts or a reflection of paranoia.

As the example above illustrates, many patients with psychotic depression have difficulty accepting that they have psychotic symptoms. For many patients, the word *psychosis* is frightening and has pejorative connotations. Thus, as my second strategy to elicit disclosure of psychotic symptoms, I use the term *irrational worries* instead of *psychosis. Irrational worries* is more acceptable to patients, and use of the term results in a greater likelihood that a patient will tell me what is on his or her mind. Rather than asking the depressed patient about psychotic symptoms, I ask whether he or she has had any irrational worries; if the answer is yes, I explore the issue further. The key here is that the term *irrational worries* allows the patient to feel comfortable explaining his or her unusual thoughts without having to worry that they will be labeled psychotic.

Psychotic Depression Versus Schizophrenia and Schizoaffective Disorder

When psychosis is prominent (particularly in young adults), differentiating schizophrenia spectrum disorders from psychotic depression can be extremely challenging. Knowledge of the course and history of a patient's depressive and psychotic symptoms is critical for making an accurate diagnosis. However, particularly in early episodes, the clinician may have difficulty ascertaining from the history whether the psychotic symptoms occur only in the context of an episode of major depression, as they do in psychotic depression, or whether they occur in the absence of mood symptoms, as in schizophrenia spectrum disorders.

A few biological differences have been documented that may assist the clinician in differentiating psychotic depression from schizophrenia and schizoaffective disorder. Patients with psychotic depression and schizophrenia differ in hypothalamic-adrenal-pituitary axis activity (see Chapter 4, "Biology") and all-night sleep electroencephalographic readings (Rothschild and Schatzberg 1993). In fact, the differential diagnosis of psychotic depression from schizophrenia and schizoaffective disorder may be the one clinical situation in which the dexamethasone suppression test may have clinical utility (American Psychiatric Association 1987).

Psychotic Depression Versus Posttraumatic Stress Disorder

Differentiating psychotic depression with a history of trauma from posttraumatic stress disorder (PTSD) with psychotic features can be quite challenging. Because PTSD frequently occurs with comorbid affective, anxiety, substance use, and personality disorders, and most commonly with major depressive disorder (Brady et al. 2000; Breslau et al. 1991), a common topic of debate has been the role of symptom overlap in the diagnosis of PTSD and other comorbid illnesses (Brady et al. 2000; Breslau et al. 1991; Franklin and Zimmerman 2001; Heffernan and Cloitre 2000). A study by Franklin and Zimmerman (2001) demonstrated that the high comorbidity of major depression among adult outpatients with PTSD was not a result of symptom overlap. Other authors have suggested a relationship among PTSD, the development of psychosis, and unipolar depression (David et al. 1999; Hamner et al. 1999; McClellan et al. 2002; Strakowski et al. 1995). Evidence also exists that connects a history of childhood abuse with the development of psychosis later in life (Beck and van der Kolk 1987; Bryer et al. 1987; Friedman and Harrison 1984; Livingston 1987; Lundberg-Love et al. 1992; Read and Argyle 1999; Swett et al. 1990); although this relationship is not entirely clear, findings suggest that patients who have been abused physically or sexually in childhood may be at higher risk of developing psychotic symptoms in the future.

Zimmerman and Mattia (1999), in an important study, demonstrated that the diagnoses of psychotic depression and PTSD are not mutually exclusive and that, in fact, they frequently co-occur in the same patient. In this study, patients with psychotic depression were four times more likely to have comorbid PTSD than were patients with nonpsychotic depression (57.9% and 15.7%, respectively).

Psychotic Depression Versus Obsessive-Compulsive Disorder

Distinguishing between psychotic depression and obsessive-compulsive disorder (OCD) can be difficult. The clinician is faced with determining whether a fixed, ruminative thought in a depressed patient represents an obsession or a delusion. Because OCD is frequently comorbid with major depression, the clinician may have difficulty in determining which disorder is primary and in deciding whether a subjectively reported abnormality of cognition represents a true delusion or an intrusive thought. Many times, the differential diagnosis is impossible. Studies that have reported the efficacy of selective serotonin reuptake inhibitor (SSRI) monotherapy in psychotic depression may have suffered from this difficult diagnostic dilemma and the lack of clear methods for distinguishing delusions from depressive and obsessive ruminations (Rothschild and Phillips 1999). From a practical standpoint for the clinician, the unusual thoughts in psychotic depression are episodic and occur only in the context of an episode of major depression. In contrast, the unusual thoughts in OCD are constantly present and usually have been present without abating for a considerable period of time.

Psychotic Depression Versus Body Dysmorphic Disorder

Differentiating psychotic depression with somatic delusions from body dysmorphic disorder with psychotic features is difficult and can have significant treatment implications. Whereas psychotic depression is usually treated with the combination of an antidepressant and an antipsychotic (Rothschild 2003), body dysmorphic disorder responds to SSRI monotherapy (Phillips 2004) and would almost never be treated with electroconvulsive therapy. Body image concerns have been correlated with poor self-esteem and depression (Bohne et al. 2002). According to DSM-IV-TR criteria, an individual with body dysmorphic disorder must display excessive concern over an imagined or slight defect, and this concern must cause substantial distress or functional impairment. In addition, the concern is not better accounted for by another mental disorder (e.g., psychotic depression, eating disorder). Similarly, in psychotic depression, the body is often a focus of delusional thinking. During depressive episodes, a patient may have a frank belief about a body part that is not consistent with reality. The patient's history may include negative medical workups or preoccupation with wanting plastic surgery. Hypochondriasis is a characteristic of psychotic depression, and distinguishing body dysmorphic disorder and other somatoform spectrum disorders from the delusions of psychotic depression may be difficult. From a practical standpoint for the clinician, the delusions in body dysmorphic disorder tend to be fixed over time, whereas those in psychotic depression occur simultaneously with the depressive episode and should subside when the acute psychotic depressive episode resolves.

Relationship to Bipolar Disorder

Several studies support a relationship between early-onset psychotic depression and bipolar disorder. Some clinicians argue that early-onset psychotic depression should be considered an initial episode of bipolar disorder until proven otherwise, but this appears to be too broad a generalization: several studies have demonstrated that some patients with early-onset psychotic depression subsequently develop bipolar disorder, whereas other patients simply experience unipolar depression (Akiskal et al. 1983; Aronson et al. 1988; Strober and Carlson 1982).

Strober and Carlson (1982) observed 60 adolescents hospitalized with unipolar major depression. They reported a 20% conversion rate to a diagnosis of bipolar disorder, predicted in part by a depressive symptom cluster consisting of mood-congruent psychotic features (75% of converters vs. 6% of nonconverters; $P<0.001$), psychomotor retardation, and rapid symptom onset. Similarly, Akiskal and colleagues (1983) observed a 20% conversion rate to a diagnosis of bipolar disorder in a follow-up of 206 outpatients with unipolar depression. Major depression with psychotic features was significantly more common (P<0.01) in patients who converted to a bipolar diagnosis (42%) than among nonconverters (15%). Furthermore, patients whose diagnosis changed from unipolar depression to bipolar illness were significantly younger at illness onset than those whose diagnosis did not change (P=0.003), with onset occurring before age 25 in 71% of the patients in the bipolar group compared with 32% of the patients in the nonbipolar group. In another study, Aronson and colleagues (1988) observed that bipolar patients, at the index episode of psychotic depression, presented at an earlier age than did patients with recurrent unipolar depression (29.7 years and 44.3 years, respectively; P=0.028). Taken together, these data suggest that bipolar disorder may often manifest as psychotic depression in adolescents or young adults. Whether, as Strober and Carlson (1982) suggest, young age is the critical variable accounting for the predictive relationship between psychoticism and bipolarity warrants further research.

Finally, clinicians interviewed 4,724 subjects with major mood disorder in three family studies on the genetics of bipolar I disorder or recurrent major depressive disorder. The presence of psychotic features during a depressive episode significantly increased the likelihood of a diagnosis of bipolar I disorder (Goes et al. 2007).

Late-Life Psychotic Depression

Although psychotic depression does occur in younger patients, the prevalence of psychotic depression may be as high as 45% in samples of older adults with major depression (Meyers and Greenberg 1986; Post 1962). In studies comparing patients with psychotic depression age 60 years or older with patients younger than age 60, the older patients had a later age at onset (Gournellis et al. 2001; Meyers and Greenberg 1986), more guilt (Baldwin 1995; Lee et al. 2003), more depressive symptoms as measured by the Hamilton Rating Scale for Depression (Baldwin 1995; Gournellis et al. 2001; Kivela and Pahkala 1989; Lee et al. 2003), and more cognitive and functional impairment (Lee et al. 2003) (see Table 5–4). A recent study (Gournellis et al. 2008) comparing delusional beliefs in patients with late-life psychotic depression (≥60 years) and in patients with young-onset psychotic depression (<60 years of age) found that those with late-onset psychotic depression exhibited more delusional beliefs of somatic and impending disaster content, including delusional beliefs of poverty, and fewer paranoid beliefs. The two groups did not differ with regard to delusional beliefs of guilt.

Published results from multicenter electroconvulsive therapy trials demonstrate that both psychotic depression and older age are well represented among patients who receive this intensive treatment (Sackeim et al. 2001). An interesting and unanswered question is whether psychotic depression with onset before age 60 and late-onset psychotic depression are different illnesses. Studies of late-life psychotic depression have suggested a relationship to dementia (Alexopoulos et al. 1993), whereas psychotic depression with onset before age 60 has been associated with a high prevalence of the later development of a manic episode, suggesting a link to bipolar disorder (Akiskal et al. 1983; Strober and Carlson 1982). Possible differences in response to treatment for earlier-onset and late-life psychotic depression have not been well studied but are a major focus of the recently completed NIMH STOP-PD (Meyers et al. 2006).

Adolescent Psychotic Depression

Psychotic depression in clinical samples of adolescents (see Table 5–5) has been associated with sexual abuse and alcohol or drug use (Haley et al. 1988; Ryan et al. 1987). In one study of homeless adolescents, psychotic symptoms were associated with depression severity, suicidal ideation, physical/sexual abuse, and drug use (Mundy et al. 1990). In

Table 5–4. Characteristics of patients with late-onset psychotic depression compared with patients with earlier-onset psychotic depression

↑ Guilt
↑ Depressive symptomatology
↑ Cognitive and functional impairment
↑ Somatic delusions
↑ Delusions of disasters

a study of 150 adolescent inpatients with major depression (Quinlan et al. 1997), delusions or hallucinations were present in 10% of the subjects. Delusions were present in 93% of the psychotic patients, and the remaining 7% had only hallucinations. Eighty percent of the patients with delusions also had hallucinations; 20% of the psychotic patients had only delusions. Similar to studies of adults discussed earlier (see subsection "Psychotic Depression Versus Posttraumatic Stress Disorder"), studies of adolescents found that inpatient adolescents with psychotic depression had a higher frequency of comorbid PTSD than did nonpsychotic depressed inpatient adolescents, and the majority of the patients with PTSD had a history of sexual abuse (Quinlan et al. 1997). The adolescents with psychotic depression also had more frequent and severe suicidal ideation than did the adolescent inpatients with nonpsychotic depression (Quinlan et al. 1997).

Psychotic Depression in Minority Populations

Atypical psychotic symptoms, which are not described in DSM-IV-TR, are frequently seen in individuals from specific cultures and religions. For example, Hispanic patients with psychotic depression are less likely to exhibit classic mood-congruent psychotic symptoms, such as depressive delusions and paranoia, and are more likely to exhibit "non-

Table 5–5. Adolescent psychotic depression

↑ Suicidal ideation
↑ Substance abuse
↑ History of physical/sexual abuse
↑ Comorbid posttraumatic stress disorder

diagnostic" symptoms, such as auditory and visual hallucinations (the latter being relatively rare in psychotic depression) (Mischoulon et al. 2005). This variation in symptoms could easily result in misdiagnosis.

African American patients with psychotic symptoms are more likely than white patients with psychotic symptoms to receive a diagnosis of schizophrenia and less likely to receive a diagnosis of psychotic depression (Strakowski et al. 1996). Even though the rates of affective syndromes are similar between the two groups, the more severe first-rank symptoms in African American patients may have influenced raters in the past to stray from using diagnostic criteria (Strakowski et al. 1996). This difference in diagnosis may also reflect a tendency to see African American patients as sicker and, conversely, white patients as less ill, thereby leading to the observed racial differences in diagnostic assignment for the groups.

Key Clinical Points

- The diagnosis of psychotic depression is frequently missed because the delusions are not recognized.
- Patients with psychotic depression are frequently guarded, making it difficult for clinicians to detect the presence of delusions.
- Family members should be involved in the assessment process.
- Nonthreatening terms, such as *irrational worries*, should be used with patients instead of *paranoia* or *psychosis*.

- Although psychotic depression can occur at any age, it may be more common in depressed patients over the age of 60.

References

Akiskal HS, Walker P, Puzantian VR, et al: Bipolar outcome in the course of depressive illness: phenomenological, familial, and pharmacologic predictors. J Affect Disord 5:115–128, 1983

Alexopoulos GS, Meyers BS, Young RC, et al: The course of geriatric depression with "reversible dementia": a controlled study. Am J Psychiatry 150:1693–1699, 1993

American Psychiatric Association: The dexamethasone suppression test: an overview of its current status in psychiatry. The APA Task Force on Laboratory Tests in Psychiatry. Am J Psychiatry 144:1253–1262, 1987

American Psychiatric Association: Diagnostic and Statistical Manual of Mental Disorders, 4th Edition, Text Revision. Washington, DC, American Psychiatric Association, 2000

Andreescu C, Mulsant BH, Peasley-Micklus C, et al; for the STOP-PD Study Group: Persisting low use of antipsychotics in the treatment of major depressive disorder with psychotic features. J Clin Psychiatry 68:194–200, 2007

Aronson TA, Shukla S, Hoff A, et al: Proposed delusional depression subtypes: preliminary evidence from a retrospective study of phenomenology and treatment course. J Affect Disord 14:69–74, 1988

Baldwin RC: Delusional depression in elderly patients: characteristics and relationship to age at onset. Int J Geriatr Psychiatry 10:981–985, 1995

Basso MR, Bornstein RA: Neuropsychological deficits in psychotic versus nonpsychotic unipolar depression. Neuropsychology 13:69–75, 1999

Beck JC, van der Kolk BA: Reports of childhood incest and current behavior of chronically hospitalized psychotic women. Am J Psychiatry 144:1474–1476, 1987

Belanoff JK, Sund B, Fleming-Fice KS, et al: Cortisol activity and cognitive changes in psychotic major depression. Am J Psychiatry 158:1612–1616, 2001

Bohne A, Keuthen NJ, Wilhelm S, et al: Prevalence of symptoms of body dysmorphic disorder and its correlates: a cross-cultural comparison. Psychosomatics 43:486–490, 2002

Brady KT, Killeen RN, Brewerton T, et al: Comorbidity of psychiatric disorders and posttraumatic stress disorder. J Clin Psychiatry 61 (suppl 7):22–32, 2000

Breslau N, Davis GC, Andreski P, et al: Traumatic events and post-traumatic stress disorder in an urban population of young adults. Arch Gen Psychiatry 48:216–222, 1991

Bryer JB, Nelson BA, Miller JB, et al: Childhood sexual and physical abuse as factors in psychiatric illness. Am J Psychiatry 144:1426–1430, 1987

Charney DS, Nelson JC: Delusional and nondelusional unipolar depression: further evidence for distinct subtypes. Am J Psychiatry 138:328–333, 1981

Coryell W, Pfohl B, Zimmerman M: The clinical and neuroendocrine features of psychotic depression. J Nerv Ment Dis 172:521–528, 1984

David D, Kutcher GS, Jackson EI, et al: Psychotic symptoms in combat-related posttraumatic stress disorder. J Clin Psychiatry 60:29–32, 1999

Frances A, Brown RP, Kocsis JH, et al: Psychotic depression: a separate entity? Am J Psychiatry 138:831–833, 1981

Franklin CL, Zimmerman M: Posttraumatic stress disorder and major depressive disorder: investigating the role of overlapping symptoms in diagnostic comorbidity. J Nerv Ment Dis 189:548–551, 2001

Friedman S, Harrison G: Sexual histories, attitudes, and behavior of schizophrenic and normal women. Arch Sex Behav 13:555–567, 1984

Gaudiano BA, Young D, Chelminski I, et al: Depressive symptom profiles and severity patterns in outpatients with psychotic vs nonpsychotic major depression. Compr Psychiatry 49:421–429, 2008

Glassman AH, Roose SP: Delusional depression: a distinct clinical entity? Arch Gen Psychiatry 38:424–427, 1981

Goes FS, Sadler B, Toolan J, et al: Psychotic features in bipolar and unipolar depression. Bipolar Disord 9:901–906, 2007

Gournellis R, Lykouras L, Fortos A, et al: Psychotic (delusional) major depression in late life: a clinical study. Int J Geriatr Psychiatry 16:1085–1091, 2001

Gournellis R, Oulis P, Christodoulou C, et al: Delusional beliefs in psychotic depression vary according to age of onset. Int J Geriatr Psychiatry 2008 (Epub ahead of print]

Haley GM, Fine S, Marriage K: Psychotic features in adolescents with major depression. J Am Acad Child Adolesc Psychiatry 27:489–493, 1988

Hamner MB, Frueh BC, Ulmer HG, et al: Psychotic features and illness severity in combat veterans with chronic posttraumatic stress disorder. Biol Psychiatry 45:846–852, 1999

Heffernan K, Cloitre M: A comparison of posttraumatic stress disorder with and without borderline personality disorder among women with a history of childhood sexual abuse: etiological and clinical characteristics. J Nerv Ment Dis 188:589–595, 2000

Jeste DV, Heaton SC, Paulsen JS, et al: Clinical and neuropsychological comparison of psychotic depression with non-psychotic depression and schizophrenia. Am J Psychiatry 153:490–496, 1996

Kivela SL, Pahkala K: Delusional depression in the elderly: a community study. Z Gerontol 22:236–241, 1989

Lee TW, Tsai SJ, Yang CH, et al: Clinical and phenomenological comparisons of delusional and non-delusional major depression in the Chinese elderly. Int J Geriatr Psychiatry 18:486–490, 2003

Livingston R: Sexually and physically abused children. J Am Acad Child Adolesc Psychiatry 26:413–415, 1987

Lundberg-Love PK, Marmion S, Ford K, et al: The long-term consequences of childhood incestuous victimization upon adult women's psychological symptomatology. J Child Sex Abus 1:81–102, 1992

Lykouras E, Malliaras D, Christodoulou GN, et al: Delusional depression: phenomenology and response to treatment. A prospective study. Acta Psychiatr Scand 73:324–329, 1986

McClellan J, McCurry C, Speltz ML, et al: Symptom factors in early onset psychotic disorders. J Am Acad Child Adolesc Psychiatry 41:791–798, 2002

Meyers BS, Greenberg R: Late-life delusional depression. J Affect Disord 11:133–137, 1986

Meyers BS, Peasley-Miklus C, Flint AJ, et al: Methodological issues in designing a randomized controlled trial for psychotic depression: the STOP-PD Study. Psychiatr Ann 36:57–64, 2006

Mischoulon D, Lagomasino I, Harmon C: Atypical psychotic symptoms in a Hispanic population: diagnostic dilemmas and implications for treatment. Psychiatry 2:38–46, 2005. Available at: http://www.psychiatrymmc.com/displayArticle.cfm?articleID=article51. Accessed June 5, 2008.

Mundy P, Robertson M, Robertson J, et al: The prevalence of psychotic symptoms in homeless adolescents. J Am Acad Child Adolesc Psychiatry 29:724–731, 1990

Nelson EB, Sax KW, Strakowski SM: Attentional performance in patients with psychotic and non-psychotic major depression and schizophrenia. Am J Psychiatry 155:137–139, 1998

Nelson JC, Bowers MB: Delusional versus unipolar depression: description and drug response. Arch Gen Psychiatry 35:1321–1328, 1978

Parker G, Hadzi-Pavlovic D, Hickie I, et al: Distinguishing psychotic and nonpsychotic melancholia. J Affect Disord 22:135–148, 1991

Phillips KA: Psychosis in body dysmorphic disorder. J Psychiatr Res 38:63–72, 2004

Post F: The Significance of Affective Symptoms in Old Age. New York, Oxford University Press, 1962

Quinlan PE, King CA, Hanna GL, et al: Psychotic versus non-psychotic depression in hospitalized adolescents. Depress Anxiety 6:40–42, 1997

Read J, Argyle N: Hallucinations, delusions, and thought disorder among adult psychiatric inpatients with a history of child abuse. Psychiatr Serv 50:1467–1472, 1999

Rothschild AJ: Challenges in the treatment of depression with psychotic features. Biol Psychiatry 53:680–690, 2003

Rothschild AJ, Phillips KA: Selective serotonin reuptake inhibitors and delusional depression. Am J Psychiatry 156:977–978, 1999

Rothschild AJ, Schatzberg AF: Psychotic depression: a newly recognized subtype. Clin Neurosci 1:75–80, 1993

Rothschild AJ, Benes F, Hebben N, et al: Relationships between brain CT scan findings and cortisol in psychotic and non-psychotic depressed patients. Biol Psychiatry 26:565–575, 1989

Rothschild AJ, Winer J, Flint AJ, et al; for the Study of Pharmacotherapy of Psychotic Depression (STOP-PD) Collaborative Study Group: Missed diagnosis of psychotic depression at 4 academic medical centers. J Clin Psychiatry 69:1293–1296, 2008

Ryan ND, Puig-Antich J, Ambrosini P, et al: The clinical picture of major depression in children and adolescents. Arch Gen Psychiatry 44:854–861, 1987

Sackeim HA, Haskett RF, Mulsant BH, et al: Continuation pharmacotherapy in the prevention of relapse following electroconvulsive therapy: a randomized controlled trial. JAMA 285:1299–1307, 2001

Schatzberg A, Posener JA, DeBattista C, et al: Neuropsychological deficits in psychotic versus non-psychotic major depression and no mental illness. Am J Psychiatry 157:1095–1100, 2000

Simpson S, Baldwin RC, Jackson A, et al: The differentiation of DSM-III-R psychotic depression in later life from nonpsychotic depression: comparisons of brain changes measured by multispectral analysis of magnetic resonance brain images, neuropsychological findings, and clinical features. Biol Psychiatry 45:193–204, 1999

Strakowski SM, Keck PE Jr, McElroy SL, et al: Chronology of comorbid and principal syndromes in first-episode psychosis. Compr Psychiatry 36:106–112, 1995

Strakowski SM, Flaum M, Amador X, et al: Racial differences in the diagnosis of psychosis. Schizophr Res 21:117–124, 1996

Strober M, Carlson G: Bipolar illness in adolescents with major depression: clinical, genetic, and psychopharmacologic predictors in a three- to four-year prospective follow-up investigation. Arch Gen Psychiatry 39:549–555, 1982

Swett C Jr, Surrey J, Cohen C: Sexual and physical abuse histories and psychiatric symptoms among male psychiatric outpatients. Am J Psychiatry 147:632–636, 1990

Zimmerman M, Mattia JI: Psychotic subtyping of major depressive disorder and posttraumatic stress disorder. J Clin Psychiatry 60:311–314, 1999

Recommended Reading

Glassman AH, Roose SP: Delusional depression: a distinct clinical entity? Arch Gen Psychiatry 38:424–427, 1981

Mischoulon D, Lagomasino I, Harmon C: Atypical psychotic symptoms in a Hispanic population: diagnostic dilemmas and implications for treatment. Psychiatry 2:38–46, 2005. Available at: http://www.psychiatrymmc.com/displayArticle.cfm?articleID=article51. Accessed June 5, 2008.

Rothschild AJ: Challenges in the treatment of depression with psychotic features. Biol Psychiatry 53:680–690, 2003

Rothschild AJ, Winer J, Flint AJ, et al; for the Study of Pharmacotherapy of Psychotic Depression (STOP-PD) Collaborative Study Group: Missed diagnosis of psychotic depression at 4 academic medical centers. J Clin Psychiatry 69:1293–1296, 2008

6

Treatment

No drugs, devices, or treatments have, as of this writing, been approved by the U.S. Food and Drug Administration specifically for the treatment of major depression with psychotic features. The American Psychiatric Association (2000), in its *Practice Guideline for the Treatment of Patients With Major Depressive Disorder,* recommends, with substantial clinical confidence, the use of an antipsychotic–antidepressant combination or electroconvulsive therapy (ECT) for the treatment of psychotic depression. In this chapter, I focus primarily on ECT and pharmacologic treatment, reviewing the current evidence base in support of their use. I also discuss continuation and maintenance treatment, review data on the use of psychotherapy for psychotic depression, and discuss the important role of the family in patient assessment and treatment. I close the chapter by summarizing the use of the somatic therapies in a clinician-friendly algorithm.

Considering Electroconvulsive Therapy Versus Medications

When treating a patient with psychotic depression, the clinician must first decide whether to prescribe medication or ECT. This question has no simple answer, and the decision depends to a large extent on the clinical situation and the patient's personal preferences. The pros and cons of medication treatment and ECT are outlined in Table 6–1.

ECT involves the application of an electrical current via scalp electrodes to induce a brief tonic-clonic seizure in anesthetized patients within a medically controlled setting. The literature comparing the relative efficacy of ECT with that of pharmacotherapies is limited by a lack of prospective, controlled trials. Meta-analysis may offer the best opportunity to synthesize published treatment outcomes; however, it is difficult to draw broad conclusions from these studies, because ECT treatment was often compared with several different combinations of medications, administered at varying dosages and for different periods of time (Rothschild 1996).

Kroessler (1985) reviewed 17 prospective and retrospective studies comprising 597 patients with psychotic depression. Response rates were 82% for ECT and 77% for the combination of a tricyclic antidepressant (TCA) and an antipsychotic, with considerably lower response rates of 51% and 34% for antidepressant monotherapy and antipsychotic monotherapy, respectively. In a larger meta-analysis, in which Parker and colleagues (1992) examined data from 44 prospective and retrospective studies published between 1959 and 1988, ECT was found to be significantly more effective than a TCA alone, with effect sizes of 2.30 and 1.16, respectively. The antidepressant–antipsychotic combination was found to have an intermediate effect size of 1.56, which was not significantly different from those of the other two treatments (Parker et al. 1992).

The early initiation of ECT within 5 days of hospital admission has been reported to shorten lengths of stay and reduce treatment costs (Olfson et al. 1998), although hospital treatment with ECT is associ-

Table 6–1. Pros and cons of medications and electroconvulsive therapy (ECT) for psychotic depression

Medications		ECT	
Pros	**Cons**	**Pros**	**Cons**
Efficacious	Medication side effects	Efficacious	Cognitive side effects
Patient acceptance	Unclear if response as fast as with ECT	Fast response	High relapse rate post-ECT
Availability			Not always available
Ease of administration			Less practical than medication
			Cost

ated with *longer* lengths of stay when treatment is not instituted rapidly (Olfson et al. 1998; Strotskopf and Horn 1992; Wilson et al. 1991).

ECT, however, does not provide a treatment alternative for the large numbers of patients who prefer pharmacologic treatment. For example, in a study of patients with psychotic depression who were recruited into a multicenter ECT study, each patient had had an average of *four* pharmacotherapy trials before entering the ECT study (Mulsant et al. 1997) (unfortunately, only 4% had actually received intensive medication treatment using an adequate dose and duration of an antidepressant and an antipsychotic).

Patients from minority ethnic groups, patients with low incomes, and patients residing in rural areas are less likely to receive ECT during a psychiatric hospitalization (Olfson et al. 1998).

Some studies suggest that ECT may be even more effective for psychotic depression than for nonpsychotic depression. An open-label retrospective study of response to an acute course of unilateral or bilateral ECT in 30 patients with unipolar psychotic depression and in 36 patients with unipolar nonpsychotic depression yielded response rates of 83% for the psychotic group and 58% for patients without psychosis (with response defined as a score <10 on the 17-item version of the Hamilton Rating Scale for Depression [Ham-D]) (Pande et al. 1990). In a larger prospective study (Petrides et al. 2001) of response to an acute course of bilateral ECT in 77 patients with unipolar psychotic depression and 176 patients with unipolar nonpsychotic depression, the rates of remission were 95% for the patients with psychotic depression and 83% for patients with nonpsychotic depression, with remission rigorously defined as 1) a score of <10 on the 24-item Ham-D measured after each of two consecutive treatments and 2) a decrease of >60% from initial scores. Improvement in symptom ratings on the Ham-D was of a greater magnitude and tended to be more rapid in the patients with psychotic depression than in those without psychosis. In a meta-analysis of studies published between 1978 and 2001, ECT was more efficacious for patients with psychotic depression than for depressed patients without psychosis (Kho et al. 2003). Finally, in a retrospective review of the records of 55 inpatients with major depression in the Netherlands, 92% of patients with psychotic depression achieved a 50% reduction in their Ham-D score, compared with 55% of nonpsychotic depressed patients (P=0.002). Fifty-eight percent of patients with psychotic depression achieved a Ham-D score of 7 or less, compared with 24% of the patients with nonpsychotic depression (P=0.01) (Birkenhager et al. 2003).

In clinical practice in the community, however, much lower remission rates have been reported than in clinical trials of ECT (Prudic et al. 2004). For example, the intent-to-treat remission rates from a large cohort of adults treated with ECT in community facilities ranged from 30% to 47% (Prudic et al. 2004). The low remission rates are of particular concern given the poor outcomes of patients whose illness does not remit with ECT (Prudic et al. 2004). The low remission rates in community practice might be explained by the fact that patients with comorbid psychiatric and medical conditions that are associated with poorer ECT outcome might represent a larger proportion of the clinical population than the patients studied in clinical trials of ECT (Prudic et al. 2004).

The Electroconvulsive Therapy Procedure

The ECT procedure consists of inducing a controlled brain seizure under anesthesia. Therefore, after obtaining written informed consent for the ECT procedure, the clinician should perform a medical evaluation of the patient to determine what special precautions may be needed during ECT anesthesia. The medical examination should include electrocardiography, measurement of electrolytes, hemoglobin and hematocrit tests, inspection of the mouth for loose teeth, and consultation with an anesthesiologist.

Current ECT devices modify ordinary electrical current, breaking it down into individual pulses in the millisecond range. The most effective electrical stimulus is a series of pulses, each 0.5–1.0 milliseconds wide, applied at a rate of between 60 and 140 pulses per second, for several seconds. The brain seizure, monitored by electroencephalography, usually lasts 25–50 seconds. Because of the anesthesia and muscle relaxants, little muscle movement occurs during the procedure. (For discussion of nursing care of the ECT patient, see Chapter 9, "Nursing Care.")

Use of ECT With Concurrent Medications

Patients with psychotic depression who are referred for ECT are often taking psychotropic medications. A question that frequently comes up is whether the medications should be discontinued. Although some practitioners have patients take psychotropic medications during a course of ECT, little evidence exists supporting the beneficial value of this practice. Furthermore, some medications might have deleterious effects if the patient continues them during ECT. These include anticonvulsants and high-dose benzodiazepines (which may hinder the effectiveness of ECT), monoamine oxidase inhibitors (which may interfere with anesthesia), lithium (which may cause neurotoxic reactions) (Penney et al. 1990; Weiner et al. 1980), and theophylline (status epilepticus) (Devanand et al. 1988). Also, after the course of ECT is completed, the patient with psychotic depression will most likely be given a different medication regimen from that administered prior to ECT (see section "Continuation and Maintenance Treatment" later in this chapter). Additionally, the effects of ECT are easier to assess when ECT is the only treatment being rendered. For all these reasons, I prefer that the patient not take any medications during the ECT treatment, except as needed for anxiety or agitation.

Frequency of ECT Treatments

The two most common regimens for ECT treatment are twice a week and three times a week. The regimen of twice a week decreases the probability of cognitive side effects but may delay improvement. Given the degree of morbidity and mortality with psychotic depression, I prefer to administer ECT three times a week.

Unilateral Versus Bilateral ECT

Although bilateral ECT (with bifrontotemporal electrode placement) has long been recognized to result in more cognitive problems than unilateral ECT (with one electrode in the right frontotemporal region and one to the right of the vertex), bilateral ECT also has long been believed to be more effective. However, the efficacy of the two types may not be very different (Sackeim et al. 1995). The matter remains the subject of considerable debate for treatment of depression in general, as well as for treatment of psychotic depression, but few studies have been done to determine whether unilateral ECT and bilateral ECT differ in efficacy. In one study, the National Institute of Mental

Health (NIMH)–sponsored Consortium for Research in ECT study, Petrides and colleagues (2001) used bilateral electrode placement at 50% above the titrated seizure threshold, with remission defined as a 24-item Ham-D score of ≤10 and a decrease of at least 60% from baseline, and observed a 95% remission rate in patients with psychotic depression. In a retrospective study in the Netherlands, Birkenhager and colleagues (2003) reviewed the medical records of patients with psychotic depression who received ECT. The researchers found that 8 of 12 patients (67%) who received unilateral ECT achieved full remission (50% decrease in Ham-D score and a final Ham-D score of ≤7); 0 of 3 patients (0%) who received unilateral ECT and then were switched to bilateral ECT achieved remission; and 7 of 11 patients (64%) who received only bilateral ECT achieved full remission.

Many practitioners consider switching a patient from unilateral to bilateral ECT if only minimal improvement is evident after six to eight treatments. Controlled clinical trials do not provide the clinician with any guidance in this situation. The clinical state of the patient (including the risk for suicide) and the increased risks of cognitive problems from use of bilateral ECT are part of this decision.

Number of ECT Treatments

A clinician cannot predict how many ECT treatments will be needed for an individual with either psychotic or nonpsychotic depression. In the Consortium for Research in ECT study (Sackeim et al. 2001), the mean number of bilateral ECT treatments administered was 10.6 for the total group of psychotic and nonpsychotic depressed patients, but the authors did not report the specific number of treatments for the psychotic subgroup. In the retrospective study from the Netherlands, the mean number of ECT treatments for patients with psychotic depression who achieved full remission (Ham-D score≤7) was 10.4 (range=4–18), and the mean number of ECT treatments for patients with psychotic depression who failed to achieve remission was 16.7 (range=10–24) (Birkenhager et al. 2003).

Clinicians should be careful not to prematurely terminate ECT when a patient is beginning to show some signs of improvement. On the other hand, little evidence is available to support the value of administering additional ECT treatments once clinical remission has occurred.

Limitations of ECT

Despite the demonstrated efficacy of ECT for the acute treatment of psychotic depression, use of this treatment has been limited by a number of considerations, including the following:

1. Preference of a large number of patients and their relatives for pharmacologic treatment, because they find both the idea and the experience of ECT, as well as the possible side effects of confusion and memory disruption (Prudic et al. 2000), unacceptable (American Psychiatric Association 2000; Flint and Rifat 1998; Parker et al. 1992)
2. Issues of accessibility (Thompson et al. 1994)
3. The cost of ECT (Olfson et al. 1998)
4. The very high rates of early relapse after successful ECT treatment (Sackeim et al. 2001; Spiker et al. 1985a) (see subsection "Maintenance Therapy After Successful ECT" later in this chapter)

As a result, pharmacologic treatment is often employed as the first-line approach except in certain situations (see Table 6–2), such as in patients with life-threatening symptoms (e.g., severe suicidal ideation, poor nourishment), patients with a history of previous good response to ECT, or older patients (Flint and Rifat 1998).

Medication Treatment of Psychotic Depression

The demonstration that ECT is effective acutely does not address the need for an easily administered pharmacotherapy to treat early relapses and avoid subsequent hospitalizations (Spiker et al. 1985b). Further-

Table 6–2. Clinical situations in which electroconvulsive therapy (ECT) should be considered as first-line treatment for psychotic depression

Life-threatening symptoms
History of previous good response to ECT
Older age

more, although ECT is very effective for the treatment of the acute episode of psychotic depression, it has been associated with high rates of early relapse (Sackeim et al. 1990, 2001), in part because it is often discontinued once the patient is better. The American Psychiatric Association (2000), in its *Practice Guideline for the Treatment of Patients With Major Depressive Disorder,* recommends, with substantial clinical confidence, the use of an antipsychotic–antidepressant combination for the medication treatment of psychotic depression. However, despite this recommendation, recent data have shown that only 5% of patients with psychotic depression receive an adequate combination of antidepressant and antipsychotic medications (Andreescu et al. 2007). These findings show a persisting low rate of adequate treatment (medication dose and duration) of psychotic depression and little change from a study published a decade earlier that also reported inadequate dose and duration of medication treatment prescribed to patients with psychotic depression (Mulsant et al. 1997).

Given the high morbidity and mortality rates associated with psychotic depression, clinicians would benefit from understanding the evidence base behind the recommendations for the use of an antidepressant–antipsychotic combination. These recommendations, initially published in 1993 (American Psychiatric Association 1993), were based in large part on two meta-analyses (Chan et al. 1987; Kroessler 1985). The authors of the meta-analyses reported that the response rate of patients with psychotic depression to TCA monotherapy was less than 40%, compared with 70%–80% response rates for those treated with a TCA–antipsychotic combination. However, of the 21 studies included in these two meta-analyses, only 1 was a randomized clinical trial conducted under double-blind controlled conditions, albeit with only 51 subjects (16–18 per cell) and no placebo control (Spiker et al. 1985b). Spiker and colleagues (1985b) compared an amitriptyline–perphenazine combination with amitriptyline alone and perphenazine alone in the treatment of patients with psychotic depression over a 5-week period. Using a 50% reduction in Ham-D and Brief Psychiatric Rating Scale (BPRS) total scores and a final Ham-D score of <12 as response criteria, these researchers noted treatment response in 14 of 18 patients (78%) treated with the combination, in contrast to 7 of 17 patients (41%) treated with amitriptyline alone and 3 of 16 (19%) patients treated with perphenazine alone. Seven of the 13 patients who failed to respond to perphenazine were not psychotic at the completion of the study but were still depressed. In this study, the mean dosages of both amitriptyline (170±45.5 mg/day) and perphenazine (55±17 mg/day) were high, in particular when one considers the drug–drug interaction between TCAs and perphenazine (TCAs tend to slow the metabolism of perphenazine, resulting in higher TCA plasma levels).

Anton and Burch (1990), in a randomized, double-blind investigation, explored whether the efficacy of an amitriptyline–perphenazine combination could be matched by monotherapy with amoxapine, an antidepressant derivative of the antipsychotic medication loxapine, with dopamine antagonist activity. A previous open-label trial with amoxapine had produced response rates of 60%–80% in the treatment of psychotic depression (Anton and Sexauer 1983). Response rates, defined by Clinical Global Impression improvement criteria, were 82% for amoxapine and 86% for the amitriptyline–perphenazine combination. Using a 50% reduction in Ham-D score as a criterion for response, Anton and Burch (1990) found response rates of 71% and 81% for amoxapine and the amitriptyline–perphenazine combination, respectively. Extrapyramidal symptoms were significantly more frequent in the patients treated with the amitriptyline–perphenazine combination than in the patients treated with amoxapine.

The randomized controlled pharmacotherapy trials of psychotic depression are summarized in Table 6–3.

Since the American Psychiatric Association's 1993 guideline was published, several large prospective studies have been done of the medication treatment of patients with psychotic depression. In two large randomized controlled trials (Rothschild et al. 2004), a combination of the selective serotonin reuptake inhibitor (SSRI) fluoxetine plus the second-generation antipsychotic olanzapine was compared with olanzapine monotherapy or placebo in 229 hospitalized patients with psychotic depression. In both studies, patients were randomly assigned to receive placebo, olanzapine (mean dosage=11.9 and 14.0 mg/day) plus placebo, or olanzapine (mean dosage=12.4 and 13.9 mg/day) plus fluoxetine (mean dosage=23.5 and 22.6 mg/day), and were followed for 8 weeks. The first trial showed a reduction in Ham-D score that was statistically greater in the combination group than in the olanzapine monotherapy group or the placebo group throughout the 8 weeks. The second trial failed to reveal any statistically significant differences between the three treatment groups, except that the Ham-D score of the combination group was statistically lower than that of the placebo group at the end of week 1. However, several aspects of the study design were biased against the fluoxetine–olanzapine combination. First, the study was powered to show a difference between olanzapine monotherapy and placebo rather than combination therapy and placebo; the resultant small sample size of the combination group limited statistical power. Second, because the study design limited fluoxetine dosing on the basis of olanzapine dosing, most subjects received only 20 mg/day of fluoxetine. If higher doses of fluoxetine had been used, greater reductions in depressive symptoms or higher response or remission rates might have resulted.

Wijkstra and colleagues (2008) reported on a double-blind, randomized controlled study of 122 hospitalized patients (ages 18–65 years) with psychotic depression at eight sites in the Netherlands. For

Table 6–3. Randomized controlled pharmacotherapy trials in patients with major depression with psychotic features

Study	*N*	Age (years) Mean	SD	Duration (weeks)	Treatment-compared dosage, mg/day (mean)	Response rate (%)
Spiker et al. 1985b	51[a]	44	13	5	Amitriptyline (217)	41
					Perphenazine (32–64)	19
					Amitriptyline (170)+perphenazine (32–64)	78
Anton and Burch 1990	46[a]	45	12	2–4	Amitriptyline (200) + perphenazine (32)	86
					Amoxapine (400)	82
Zanardi et al. 1996	46[a]	54	13	6	Sertraline (150)	75
					Paroxetine (50)	46
Müller-Siecheneder et al. 1998	38[a]	46	—	5	Haloperidol (9) + amitriptyline (180) Risperidone (6.9)	70 and 51 51 and 37
Zanardi et al. 1998	72[a]	47	10	6	Fluvoxamine (300)	80
					Fluvoxamine (300)+pindolol (7.5)	81

Table 6–3. Randomized controlled pharmacotherapy trials in patients with major depression with psychotic features *(continued)*

Study	*N*	Age (years) Mean	SD	Duration (weeks)	Treatment-compared dosage, mg/day (mean)	Response rate (%)
Zanardi et al. 2000	28[a]	51	11	6	Fluvoxamine (300)	79
					Venlafaxine (300)	58
Mulsant et al. 2001	36[a]	72	8	4–18	Nortriptyline (100 ng/mL; range = 50–150 ng/mL)	44
					Nortriptyline (100 ng/mL; range = 50–150 ng/mL)+ perphenazine (8–24)	50
Rothschild et al. 2004						
Trial 1	124[a]	40.7	12.6	8	Olanzapine (11.9)	35
					Olanzapine+fluoxetine (12.4/23.5)	64
					Placebo	28

Table 6–3. Randomized controlled pharmacotherapy trials in patients with major depression with psychotic features *(continued)*

Study	*N*	Age (years) Mean	Age (years) SD	Duration (weeks)	Treatment-compared dosage, mg/day (mean)	Response rate (%)
Rothschild et al. 2004 *(continued)*						
Trial 2	125[a]	4.1	10.4	8	Olanzapine (14.0)	36
					Olanzapine+fluoxetine (13.9/22.6)	48
					Placebo	32
Meyers et al. 2008	259[b]	58	18	12	Olanzapine (14.7)	49[c]
					Olanzapine+sertraline (14.3/169)	67[c]
Wijkstra et al. 2008	122[a]	50.6	10.9	7	Imipramine (200–300 ng/mL)	42
					Venlafaxine (up to 375 mg)	39
					Venlafaxine (up to 375 mg) +quetiapine (up to 600 mg)	41

[a]Hospitalized at entry into study. [b]69% hospitalized at entry into study. [c]Remission rate of subjects completing the study.

7 weeks, 42 patients were treated with imipramine (dose adjusted to adequate plasma levels of 200–300 ng/mL), 39 with venlafaxine (maximum = 375 mg/day), and 41 with a venlafaxine–quetiapine combination (maximum 375 mg/day venlafaxine and 600 mg/day quetiapine). The primary outcome measure was a response on the Ham-D (≥50% decrease and final score ≤14). Remission was defined as a final Ham-D score of 7 or less. Response rates for patients treated with imipramine, venlafaxine, and venlafaxine–quetiapine were 22/42 (52.4%), 13/39 (33.3%), and 27/41 (65.9%), respectively. For the primary outcome measure of response, the venlafaxine–quetiapine combination was statistically significantly more effective than venlafaxine; there were no statistically significant differences in the response rates between venlafaxine–quetiapine and imipramine, or between imipramine and venlafaxine. Remission rates indicated that the venlafaxine–quetiapine combination (17/41, 41.5%) was statistically significantly more effective than imipramine (9/42, 21.4%), but was not statistically significantly different from venlafaxine (11/39, 28.2%). In addition, there was no significant difference between imipramine and venlafaxine. Wijkstra and colleagues (2008) concluded that the venlafaxine–quetiapine combination was more effective than venlafaxine alone on the primary outcome measure (response) and was well tolerated by patients.

On the basis of results from the recently completed NIMH Study of the Pharmacotherapy of Psychotic Depression (STOP-PD), Meyers and colleagues (2008) reported that the combination of an antidepressant (sertraline) and an atypical antipsychotic medication (olanzapine) was more efficacious than monotherapy with the atypical antipsychotic. The study included 259 subjects with psychotic depression; 142 were age 60 years or older and 117 were younger than 60. Of these subjects, 129 were randomly assigned to receive combination treatment (sertraline + olanzapine), and 130 were randomly assigned to receive olanzapine plus placebo. Remission was defined as a Ham-D score of ≤10 at two consecutive assessments and no delusions, as classified by a Schedule for Affective Disorders and Schizophrenia delusion severity score of

1 at the second assessment when the 2-week Ham-D depression remission criterion was met. Subjects who achieved a Ham-D score of ≤10 for the first time at week 12 were assessed again at week 13 to determine whether the 2-week duration criterion for remission was met. The dosing regimen in the STOP-PD was as follows: 1) start sertraline/placebo at a dose of 50 mg and olanzapine at a dose of 5 mg as tolerated (frail elderly subjects initially received 2.5 mg of olanzapine and 25 mg of sertraline/placebo); 2) increase the dosage of sertraline/placebo by 50 mg/day and of olanzapine by 5 mg/day every 3 days as tolerated; 3) attempt to reach minimum doses of 100 mg/day of sertraline or placebo and 10 mg/day of olanzapine before the end of week 1; 4) increase doses to 150 mg/day of sertraline or placebo and 15 mg/day of olanzapine during week 2; 5) allow use of sertraline/placebo at 200 mg/day and olanzapine at 20 mg/day for residual symptoms beginning in week 3; and 6) allow slower titration or temporary dose reductions of one or both medications if side effects are suspected; however, subsequent dose increases were required to attempt to achieve minimum target doses of 150 mg/day of sertraline or placebo and 15 mg/day of olanzapine.

Meyers et al. (2008), in the STOP-PD, reported that 67% of the study completers who received the olanzapine–sertraline combination achieved remission by week 12, compared with only 49% of study completers who received olanzapine monotherapy ($\chi^2 = 10.42$, $df = 1$, $P = 0.04$). An analysis of all randomly assigned subjects found that the combination of olanzapine and sertraline was associated with a greater frequency of remission (42% of 129 subjects) than was olanzapine monotherapy (24% of 130 subjects) ($\chi^2 = 9.53$, $df = 1$, $P = 0.002$). The superior efficacy of olanzapine plus sertraline increased over time (OR = 1.28, 95% CI = 1.12–1.47, $P < 0.001$). Separation began at week 8 and continued through week 12. Remission rates in the young adult and geriatric samples were comparable. The rates and severity of adverse events were similar in the older and younger patients, and the older subjects did not demonstrate poorer overall tolerability. The older subjects were more likely than younger subjects to experience pedal edema, but the older subjects were no more likely to experience falls, experience sedation/somnolence, or have greater extrapyramidal symptoms. Both age groups experienced significant increases in weight, triglycerides, and cholesterol levels. However, older patients gained less weight, which may be partially explained by their lower cumulative olanzapine dose (Smith et al. 2008). Fasting glucose levels increased significantly only in younger adults.

Selection of an Antidepressant–Antipsychotic Combination

Four antidepressant–antipsychotic combinations have been shown to be effective in randomized controlled clinical trials of patients with psychotic depression. These combinations include amitriptyline plus perphenazine (Spiker et al. 1985b), fluoxetine plus olanzapine (Rothschild et al. 2004), sertraline plus olanzapine (Meyers et al. 2008), and venlafaxine plus quetiapine (Wijkstra et al. 2008) (see Table 6–4). Because other combinations of antidepressants and antipsychotics have not been studied, I recommend using these four combinations until there is evidence that other combinations are effective. If a patient does not respond to trials of one or two of these combinations, the clinician should seriously consider ECT.

Augmentation Strategies

Lithium augmentation of antidepressants is a well-known strategy for treating nonpsychotic depression, particularly for individuals who respond only partially to antidepressants (Bauer and Dopfmer 1999). However, lithium augmentation has not been adequately studied in the treatment of psychotic depression. In three small, uncontrolled studies, lithium augmentation of an antidepressant–antipsychotic combination appeared to improve efficacy, particularly in bipolar patients. In the first study, lithium augmentation of a TCA and an older typical an-

Table 6–4. Combinations of antidepressant and antipsychotic medications with demonstrated efficacy in psychotic depression in randomized controlled clinical trials

Study	Sample size	Antidepressant	Antipsychotic
Spiker et al. 1985b	51	Amitriptyline	Perphenazine
Rothschild et al. 2004[a]	249	Fluoxetine	Olanzapine
Meyers et al. 2008	259	Sertraline	Olanzapine
Wijkstra et al. 2008	122	Venlafaxine	Quetiapine

[a]Only study with a placebo control group.

tipsychotic medication was shown to be efficacious for psychotic depression (Price et al. 1983). In a retrospective chart review of patients whose psychotic depression was refractory to treatment with desipramine plus perphenazine (12–64 mg) or haloperidol (4–20 mg), 8 of 9 patients with bipolar psychotic depression, but only 3 of 12 patients with unipolar psychotic depression, recovered when lithium (600–1,200 mg/day) was added (Fisher exact test, $P=0.003$) (Nelson and Mazure 1986). Similarly, in a study of 8 patients who had not responded to 5 weeks of treatment with a fluoxetine–perphenazine combination, 3 of 3 patients with bipolar psychotic depression responded to lithium augmentation, in contrast to none of the 5 patients with unipolar psychotic depression ($P<0.01$) (Rothschild et al. 1993). The use of other augmentation strategies or the use of lithium augmentation with other combinations of antidepressant and antipsychotic medications has not been studied.

Effectiveness of Antidepressant Monotherapy

Only two randomized clinical trials have compared antidepressant monotherapy with an antidepressant–antipsychotic combination. Results from Spiker and colleagues' (1985b) study, discussed previously in the section "Medication Treatment of Psychotic Depression," indicated that the antidepressant–antipsychotic combination was superior to antidepressant monotherapy. In contrast, Mulsant and colleagues (2001), in a study of older patients (mean age=72 years) with psychotic depression, observed no difference between antidepressant monotherapy and the antidepressant–antipsychotic combination. In fact, the response was mediocre for both groups. Mulsant and colleagues' (2001) study was a double-blind trial comparing the tolerability and efficacy of nortriptyline plus perphenazine versus nortriptyline plus placebo in a group of older inpatients who presented with a major depressive episode with psychotic features. Fifty-two patients started receiving, on an open basis, nortriptyline that was titrated to yield a therapeutic plasma level (target = 100 ng/mL; range=50–150 ng/mL). Once the plasma nortriptyline level was within the therapeutic range, subjects were randomly assigned to the addition of perphenazine (n=17) or placebo (n=19). The dosage of perphenazine or placebo was titrated up to a maximum of 24 mg/day (mean dosage=18.9 mg/day), until patients showed therapeutic response or until extrapyramidal side effects were detected. Thirty patients completed the study receiving nortriptyline for at least 4 weeks combined with either perphenazine (n=14) or placebo (n=16) for at least 2 weeks. No statistical differences were observed on the Ham-D or on the Psychoticism subscale of the BPRS between the two groups. Rates of response to the nortriptyline–perphenazine combination (50%) and nortriptyline monotherapy (44%) did not statistically differ among the 30 patients who completed treatment (P=0.99).

A meta-analysis of these two studies (Wijkstra et al. 2006) did not show a statistically significant difference between a TCA plus an antipsychotic and a TCA alone (relative risk [RR]=1.44, 95% CI=0.86–2.41; P=0.16), leading Wijkstra and colleagues to conclude that either antidepressant monotherapy or an antidepressant–antipsychotic combination was an appropriate pharmacotherapy option for psychotic depression. I disagree with this conclusion. In their study, Spiker and colleagues (1985b) found that the amitriptyline–perphenazine combination was significantly more efficacious than amitriptyline monotherapy. Combining these data with those of Mulsant and colleagues (2001), who used a different study design and had mediocre results on both nortriptyline monotherapy and the nortriptyline–perphenazine combination, obscures the finding of Spiker and colleagues' study.

In a post hoc analysis (Birkenhager et al. 2008) of two randomized controlled clinical trials of imipramine monotherapy with plasma level–targeted dosing and response (defined as at least a 50% decrease in Ham-D score), 55% of patients with mood-congruent psychotic depression responded, compared with 39% of depressed patients without psychotic features (P=0.09). Rates of remission, defined as at least a 50% decrease in Ham-D score and a final Ham-D score of ≤7, for psychotic depressed patients (25%) were not statistically different from those for nonpsychotic depressed patients (24%) (P=0.94).

In a series of studies published during the 1990s, an Italian research group reported marked improvement of inpatients with psychotic depression treated with SSRI monotherapy, including fluvoxamine, paroxetine, and sertraline (Bellini et al. 1994; Gatti et al. 1996; Zanardi et al. 1996, 1998, 2000). In these studies, patients' response rates to SSRI monotherapy were comparable to the response rates observed in other studies with ECT or with a combination of TCA and antipsychotic. These response rates are remarkably high given the relatively short duration of treatment (i.e., ≤6 weeks). These studies have been criticized, however, because of the lack of a placebo control, concerns regarding the diagnostic inclusion criteria, and the validity of the scales used for evaluation of response (Rothschild and Phillips 1999). Also, the results have not been replicated by another research group. In an 8-week open-label study using sertraline monotherapy (mean dosage= 177 mg/day) for psychotic depression, Simpson and colleagues (2003) failed to replicate these findings.

Over the years, there have been case reports of an association between TCA or SSRI monotherapy and an exacerbation of psychotic symptoms in patients with unipolar psychotic depression (Narayan et al. 1995; Nelson et al. 1979). In a recent analysis of 20 studies of psychotic depression, Kantrowitz and Tampi (2008) reported that 15 (8 of whom were taking TCAs) of 177 subjects (8.5%) receiving antidepressant monotherapy had an exacerbation of psychosis, whereas only 2 of 129 subjects (1.6%) receiving either antipsychotic or combination treatment had an exacerbation of psychosis. Thus, TCA monotherapy was statistically significantly more likely to be temporally associated with an exacerbation of psychosis (P=0.007) than was antipsychotic monotherapy or the combination of an antidepressant and an antipsychotic.

Taken together, the studies of antidepressant monotherapy provide little evidence that antidepressants by themselves are as efficacious as the combination of antidepressant plus antipsychotic. Furthermore, antidepressant monotherapy may carry some risk of exacerbating the psychotic symptoms in psychotic depression.

Effectiveness of Antipsychotic Monotherapy

Five randomized clinical trials have been done comparing antipsychotic monotherapy with an antidepressant–antipsychotic combination (Meyers et al. 2008; Müller-Siecheneder et al. 1998; Rothschild et al. 2004 [two studies]; Spiker et al. 1985b). Four of five studies found a significantly greater efficacy of the combination treatment. A meta-analysis (Wijkstra et al. 2006) of three of the studies (Rothschild et al. 2004 [two studies]; Spiker et al. 1985b) showed a statistically significant difference favoring the combination compared with antipsychotic monotherapy (RR=1.92, 95% CI=1.32–2.80; P=0.0007). The studies by Spiker, Rothschild, and Meyers and their respective colleagues (all exclusively involving patients with psychotic depression) were discussed previously in this chapter (see section "Medication Treatment of Psychotic Depression"). In the study by Müller-Siecheneder and colleagues (1998), risperidone monotherapy was compared with the combination of amitriptyline plus haloperidol in a 6-week double-blind study in patients with psychotic depression (n=38), as well as patients with schizoaffective disorder (n=66) and schizophrenia-spectrum disorder with major depressive symptoms (n=19). Compared with monotherapy, combination therapy resulted in a significantly greater decrease in scores on the Bech-Rafaelsen Melancholia Scale (70% vs. 51%) and the Positive and Negative Syndrome Scale for Schizophrenia derived from the BPRS (51% vs. 37%). However, given the mixed sample, it is not clear to what extent these results apply specifically to patients with psychotic depression. Taken together, these five studies provide little support for using antipsychotic monotherapy instead of an antidepressant–antipsychotic combination.

Treatment of Bipolar Disorder Patients Who Have Psychotic Depression

No studies have specifically addressed the treatment of patients with bipolar disorder who have an episode of depression with psychotic features. Studies of patients with psychotic depression have generally focused on unipolar psychotic depression, whereas studies of patients with bipolar disorder have focused on patients in the manic phase or depressed phase but not in a depressed phase with psychotic features. Consequently, the clinician must extrapolate from studies of patients with unipolar psychotic depression for guidance regarding the optimal treatment of patients with bipolar disorder who are experiencing a depressed phase with psychotic features.

In two uncontrolled studies, lithium augmentation of an antipsychotic and of an antidepressant was found to be more efficacious for bipolar psychotic depression than for unipolar psychotic depression. In a retrospective chart review of patients with psychotic depression that was refractory to treatment with desipramine plus 12–64 mg of perphenazine or 4–20 mg of haloperidol, 8 of 9 patients with bipolar psychotic depression, but only 3 of 12 patients with unipolar psychotic depression, recovered when lithium (600–1,200 mg/day) was added (Fisher exact test, P=0.003) (Nelson and Mazure 1986). Similarly, in a study from our group (Rothschild et al. 1993), of 8 patients who did not respond to 5 weeks of treatment with the combination of fluoxetine and perphenazine, 3 of 3 patients with bipolar psychotic depression responded to lithium augmentation, in contrast to 0 of 5 patients with unipolar psychotic depression ($P<0.01$). As in unipolar psychotic depression, ECT is an effective treatment for bipolar psychotic depression (Sachs et al. 2000).

Continuation and Maintenance Treatment

Determining the optimal continuation and maintenance therapy for psychotic depression is of special concern due to the high rate of relapse observed in naturalistic follow-up studies of psychotic depression, including relapse after ECT (Aronson et al. 1987; Sackeim et al. 1990, 2001). Other concerns include a relapsing or chronic course (Murphy 1983), high mortality rates (Murphy 1983; Vythilingam et al. 2003), a high risk of extrapyramidal symptoms and tardive dyskinesia with first-generation antipsychotics (Dolder and Jeste 2003), an increased use of health care services (Johnson et al. 1991), and a high rate of disability (Johnson et al. 1991).

Continuation and Maintenance Pharmacotherapy

The studies of continuation or maintenance pharmacotherapy for psychotic depression are summarized in Table 6–5. Only one randomized controlled trial of continuation pharmacotherapy for psychotic depression has been published (Meyers et al. 2001). In this study, the benefits and risks of combination pharmacotherapy with nortriptyline or sertraline plus perphenazine were compared with those of antidepressant monotherapy with nortriptyline or sertraline during a 26-week period in 28 older patients with psychotic depression who had achieved symptom remission after being treated with ECT. Patients received a therapeutic dose of nortriptyline, or sertraline if nortriptyline was contraindicated, and were randomly assigned to receive perphenazine (mean dose=10.3 mg/day; range=8–24 mg/day) or placebo. Overall,

Table 6–5. Studies of continuation or maintenance pharmacotherapy for psychotic depression

Study	Study type	*N*	Age, years (SD)	Medication	Duration of follow-up	Relapse rate
Flint and Rifat 1998	Open[a]	19 (vs. 68)	74.7 (5.2) vs. 73.5 (6.6)	Nortriptyline (50–150 ng/mL)	2 years	47% vs. 15% P=0.005
Meyers et al. 2001	RCT[b]	28	72.2 (8.5)	Nortriptyline (50–150 ng/mL) + perphenazine 12–16 mg/day	26 weeks	15% on monotherapy vs. 33% on combination; no statistically significant difference
Rothschild and Duval 2003	Open	30	42.4 (11.7)	Fluoxetine 20–40 mg/day + perphenazine 32 mg/day	4 months of combination therapy followed by 8 months of monotherapy with fluoxetine	73% exhibited no signs of relapse over next 11 months; 27% relapsed when perphenazine was tapered after 4 months

Note. RCT = randomized clinical trial.
[a]Psychotic vs. nonpsychotic major depressive disorder.
[b]Monotherapy with tricyclic antidepressant vs. combination therapy in psychotic depression.

25% of the patients relapsed during the 26-week trial: 33% in the combination therapy group and 15% in the monotherapy group. The difference was not statistically significant because of the small sample size. Patients in the combination group were more likely to develop medication side effects, including a 43% incidence of tardive dyskinesia after 6 months of perphenazine treatment, even though none of the subjects had been exposed to prolonged antipsychotic treatment before entering the study.

In an open-label maintenance study, Rothschild and Duval (2003) assessed the effect of discontinuing antipsychotic medication in patients with psychotic depression. The study included 30 patients who had received the diagnosis of unipolar major depression with psychotic features and who responded to the combination of fluoxetine and perphenazine. If the patient was stable for 4 months on the combination, the perphenazine was then gradually tapered off. Impending relapse was defined as any of the following: 1) symptoms meeting DSM-IV (American Psychiatric Association 1994) criteria for major depression (with or without psychotic features); 2) a total Ham-D score of 17 or more; or 3) the presence of any psychotic symptoms. After tapering of the perphenazine following 4 months of treatment with fluoxetine and perphenazine, 22 of the 30 patients (73%) did not exhibit signs of relapse over the next 11 months while remaining on fluoxetine monotherapy. Patients who showed signs of relapse after antipsychotic taper were more likely to have had a longer duration of the current episode, to have had a history of more frequent past episodes, and to be younger (under age 30 years).

In another open-label maintenance study, Flint and Rifat (1998) followed a group of patients older than age 60 with major depression with or without psychotic features for 2 years after remission of their index episode. The 68 patients with nonpsychotic depression were maintained on the treatment to which they had responded in the acute phase (i.e., a therapeutic dose of nortriptyline with or without lithium augmentation), whereas 15 of the 19 patients in the psychotic depression group were treated with ECT and then switched to nortriptyline. (The 4 patients who declined ECT were treated with nortriptyline and perphenazine, and 2 of them needed further augmentation with lithium.) For patients who were treated acutely with perphenazine, the antipsychotic was discontinued by tapering the dose during a 4-week period starting 16 weeks after the start of remission. Patients with psychotic depression were significantly more likely to suffer a relapse or a recurrence than were those with nonpsychotic depression (47% and 15%, respectively; P=0.005).

The results of these various studies seem to support continuing the antidepressant–antipsychotic combination in patients with psychotic depression who have responded to the combination. The next question concerns how long this treatment should continue. Based on findings from the studies discussed above, my practice is to leave a patient on the antidepressant–antipsychotic combination to which he or she has responded for an additional 4 months. After 4 months, if the patient has remained in remission, I begin a gradual taper of the antipsychotic medication while having the patient continue taking the antidepressant. If the patient is having significant side effects (e.g., signs of tardive dyskinesia with an older antipsychotic medication or metabolic syndrome symptoms with a newer antipsychotic agent), I may start the taper before 4 months have passed. On the other hand, if the patient is having no side effects and/or is still symptomatic, I may wait beyond 4 months to begin the taper of the antipsychotic medication. In these cases, I usually have the patient continue taking the antidepressant indefinitely, given the high rate of relapse in psychotic depression and the significant morbidity and mortality associated with relapses.

Maintenance Therapy After Successful ECT

Unfortunately, despite the demonstrated efficacy of ECT in the acute episode of psychotic depression, a rapid increase in depressive symptoms often occurs within days to weeks after the completion of a course of ECT (Prudic et al. 2004; Sackeim et al. 1993, 2001). Also, much lower remission rates following ECT (i.e., 30%–47%) are reported in community settings than in academic medical centers (Prudic et al. 2004).

In a randomized, double-blind study of maintenance pharmacotherapy of psychotic depression after successful ECT (Sackeim et al. 2001), patients were assigned to maintenance therapy with nortriptyline monotherapy, nortriptyline plus lithium, or placebo. Fifty percent of the patients experienced relapse within 6 months. Although the authors did not report the specific relapse rate for each maintenance therapy for psychotic depression, in the overall group of psychotic and nonpsychotic depressed patients, the relapse rate was statistically significantly lower with the combination of nortriptyline and lithium than with nortriptyline monotherapy or placebo.

Thus, the clinician is faced with a dilemma. Although the recently recovered patient with psychotic depression should be treated with maintenance pharmacotherapy after successful ECT, the clinician must decide what treatment to use. A common scenario is the following: A patient with psychotic depression taking antidepressant A and antipsychotic B relapses and is admitted to a psychiatric inpatient unit. The patient receives ECT and improves, and the clinician wants to prescribe maintenance pharmacotherapy. The only treatments known to be successful with the patient are ECT and the combination of medications A and B. Does the clinician prescribe medications A and B again? Most clinicians would not, arguing that the patient relapsed while taking A and B. Maintenance ECT is an option, but it is not as practical as taking medications and is more costly and not always available. In addition, the number and frequency of maintenance ECT treatments have not been studied in psychotic depression. What often ends up happening is that the clinician tries a combination of antidepressant and antipsychotic medications that the patient has not taken before and hopes that the regimen will prevent the patient from relapsing.

Psychotherapy for Patients With Psychotic Depression

Unfortunately, development in the area of psychotherapy for psychotic depression is currently lacking, because patients with psychotic features have historically been excluded from trials of psychotherapy for depression. Given the rates of morbidity and mortality associated with psychotic depression, psychosocial treatments for patients with psychotic depression are urgently needed. In one recent approach, Gaudiano and Herbert (2006) tested the efficacy of *acceptance and commitment therapy* (ACT), a modified version of cognitive-behavioral therapy, in a sample of hospitalized patients with psychotic symptoms, which included 18 patients with psychotic depression. In this pilot trial, 18 patients with psychotic depression were randomly assigned to enhanced treatment as usual (ETAU) ($n=9$) or ETAU plus individual ACT sessions ($n=9$); the number of ACT sessions varied based on the patient's length of stay (the average was three sessions). The patients receiving ACT were taught to increase their acceptance of unavoidable distress, to simply notice their psychotic symptoms without treating them as either true or false, and to identify and work toward personally valued goals despite their symptoms (Bach et al. 2006).

In a secondary analysis of the 18 patients with psychotic depression (9 assigned to the ETAU+ACT group and 9 assigned to the ETAU-only group), the average length of hospital stay was 9 (±8) days (Guadiano et al. 2007). The results indicated that 44% of the patients with psychotic depression in the ACT group showed clinically significant improvement by discharge (≥2 SD change from before to after treatment) on BPRS total scores compared with 0% of the ETAU-only group ($\chi^2=5.14$, $P<0.05$). The rates of clinically significant change on the BPRS mood symptoms subscale were 70% in the ACT group and 30% in the ETAU-only group ($\chi^2=3.60$, $P=0.058$). No significant differences were found between the two groups' rates of clinically significant change on the BPRS positive symptoms subscale.

Although these findings are intriguing, the longer-term effects of the ACT intervention on symptoms and functioning are not known. It will be important for future research to evaluate the efficacy of ACT in larger samples of patients with psychotic depression to ascertain whether it can provide an additional therapeutic modality to medications or ECT.

Family Support and Involvement

The support and involvement of the patient's family play a critical role in both the assessment and the treatment of the person with psychotic depression.

Assessment

As discussed in Chapter 5 ("Diagnosis and Assessment"), a family member often plays a key role in helping the clinician to diagnose psychotic depression. Because the person with psychotic depression often keeps his or her delusional thoughts private, the family plays a critical role as observers of any unusual thoughts or behaviors that the patient may exhibit. Although patients with psychotic depression are often brought to treatment by a family member, if they are not, it is extremely important that the clinician attempt to obtain permission from the patient to involve a family member.

Treatment

Family members play an important role during the treatment of their loved one with psychotic depression. Therefore, family members need to be educated about psychotic depression, particularly the fact that although it is a treatable illness, morbidity and mortality are significant concerns. Education regarding the treatment being rendered and its side effects is also important. Because in today's health care environment, patients are often discharged from the inpatient setting while still having significant symptoms, the family also needs to be instructed in the importance of follow-up care after discharge and the signs of worsening.

Return to Work and Reintegration Into the Community

Although the person who has an episode of psychotic depression can expect to make a full recovery and return to full occupational and social functioning in the community, the rate at which recovery will happen is highly variable. Some patients respond quickly to treatment, with fast resolution of depressive and psychotic symptoms, whereas other patients may require a significantly longer period of time for full recovery. In general, the return to functioning in patients with psychotic depression is slower than in patients with nonpsychotic depression but significantly faster than in patients with schizophrenia. In my experience, patients who are likely to return to full social and occupational functioning quickly are those who are recovering from their first episode, have a good response to the somatic treatment prescribed (whether pharmacotherapy or ECT), are between the ages of 30 and 65 years, and have good premorbid functioning. For these people, a gradual return to normal activities (including work) may occur once the person is in remission. I usually recommend a gradual increase in stressors such as work (e.g., a patient may return to part-time work and gradually increase the hours to full time).

For patients who are discharged despite having a more gradual resolution of symptoms or a partial remission of symptoms, more treatment will need to take place outside of the inpatient setting. These patients may require a combination of outpatient treatment, day treatment programs, and occupational and rehabilitation therapy (see Chapter 8, "Treatment Settings"). These patients are more likely to have had several previous episodes, to be younger than age 30 or older than age 65, and to have had a poorer premorbid level of functioning.

In either scenario outlined above, the clinician, patient, and family need to be mindful of the possibility of the return of depressive and psychotic symptoms, particularly during the 12 months after the episode. Close monitoring of the patient by the clinician, with the family's help, will enable an earlier recognition of changes in the patient's mood, cognition, or behavior that may indicate impending relapse.

Algorithm for the Somatic Treatment of Psychotic Depression

The most effective somatic treatments for psychotic depression are an antidepressant–antipsychotic combination and ECT. On the basis of the available studies to date, I have designed an algorithm, shown in Figure 6–1, to help guide the clinician in the use of the available somatic treatments.

Key Clinical Points

- The most effective somatic treatments for psychotic depression are ECT and an antidepressant–antipsychotic combination.
- Studies indicate a high relapse rate of psychotic depression, even after a good response to ECT.
- Patients with psychotic depression need continued somatic treatment during the continuation and maintenance phase of treatment.
- Studies indicate that when patients with psychotic depression are treated with medication, they frequently do not receive an adequate dose or duration of the combination of an antidepressant and an antipsychotic.
- A modified version of cognitive-behavioral therapy is being studied for the treatment of psychotic depression.
- Support and involvement of the family of the patient with psychotic depression play a critical role in the accurate assessment and treatment of the patient.

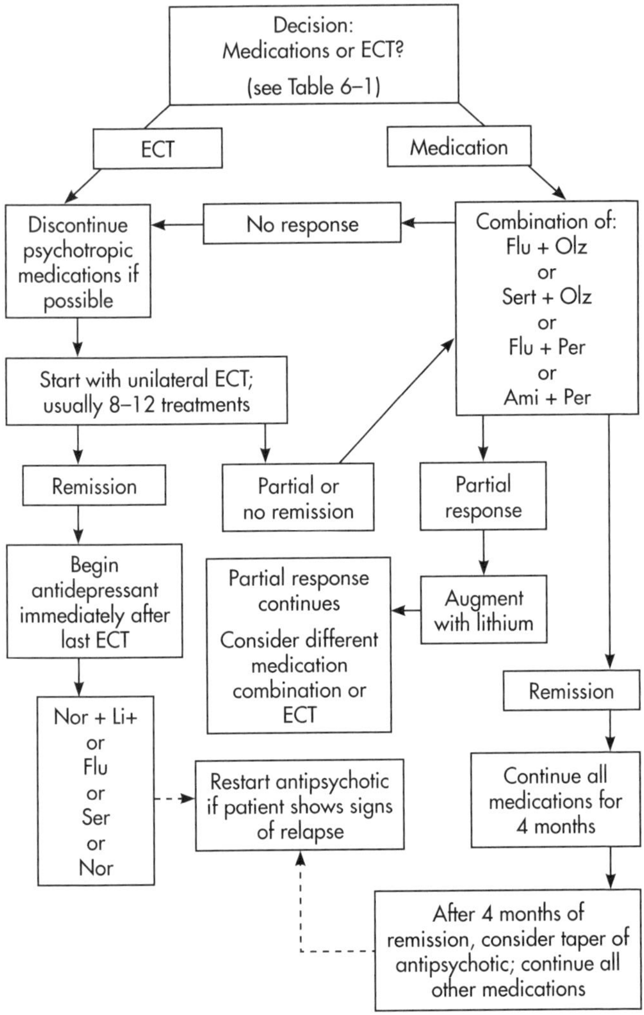

Figure 6–1. Algorithm for somatic treatment of psychotic depression.

Ami=amitriptyline; ECT=electroconvulsive therapy; Flu=fluoxetine; Li^+=lithium carbonate; Nor=nortriptyline; Olz=olanzapine; Per = perphenazine; Ser=sertraline.

References

American Psychiatric Association: Practice guideline for major depressive disorder in adults. Am J Psychiatry 150 (suppl 4):1–26, 1993

American Psychiatric Association: Practice Guideline for the Treatment of Patients With Major Depressive Disorder, 2nd Edition. Washington, DC, American Psychiatric Association, 2000

Andreescu C, Mulsant BH, Peasley-Micklus C, et al; for the Study of Pharmacotherapy of Psychotic Depression (STOP-PD) Collaborative Study Group: Persisting low use of antipsychotics in the treatment of major depressive disorder with psychotic features. J Clin Psychiatry 68:194–200, 2007

Anton RF Jr, Burch EA Jr: Amoxapine versus amitriptyline combined with perphenazine in the treatment of psychotic depression. Am J Psychiatry 147:1203–1208, 1990

Anton RF, Sexauer JD: Efficacy of amoxapine in psychotic depression. Am J Psychiatry 140:1344–1347, 1983

Aronson TA, Shukla S, Hoff A: Continuation therapy after ECT for delusional depression: a naturalistic study of prophylactic treatments and relapse. Convuls Ther 3:251–259, 1987

Bach P, Gaudiano BA, Pankey J, et al: Acceptance, mindfulness, values and psychosis: applying Acceptance and Commitment Therapy (ACT) to the chronically mentally ill, in Mindfulness-Based Treatment Approaches: Clinician's Guide to Evidence Base and Applications. Edited by Baer RA. New York, Academic Press, 2006, pp 93–116

Bauer M, Dopfmer S: Lithium augmentation in treatment-resistant depression: meta-analysis of placebo-controlled trials. J Clin Psychopharmacol 19:427–434, 1999

Bellini L, Gasperini M, Gatti L, et al: A double blind study with fluvoxamine vs. desipramine combined with placebo or haloperidol in delusional depression, in Critical Issues in the Treatment of Affective Disorders. Edited by Langer S, Brunello NR, Racagni G. Basel, S Karger, 1994, pp 32–36

Birkenhager TK, Pluijims EM, Lucius SAP: ECT response in delusional versus non-delusional depressed inpatients. J Affect Disord 74:191–195, 2003

Birkenhager TK, van den Broek WW, Mulder PG, et al: Efficacy of imipramine in psychotic versus nonpsychotic depression. J Clin Psychopharmacol 28:166–170, 2008

Chan CH, Janiak PG, Davis JM, et al: Response of psychotic and nonpsychotic depressed patients to tricyclic antidepressants. J Clin Psychiatry 48:197–200, 1987

Devanand DP, Decina P, Sackeim HA, et al: Status epilepticus following ECT in a patient receiving theophylline (letter). J Clin Psychopharmacol 8:153, 1988

Dolder CR, Jeste DV: Incidence of tardive dyskinesia with typical versus atypical anti-psychotics in very high risk patients. Biol Psychiatry 53:1142–1145, 2003

Flint AJ, Rifat SL: The treatment of psychotic depression in later life: a comparison of pharmacotherapy and ECT. J Geriatr Psychiatry 13:23–28, 1998

Gatti F, Bellini L, Gasperini M, et al: Fluvoxamine alone in the treatment of delusional depression. Am J Psychiatry 153:414–416, 1996

Gaudiano BA, Herbert JD: Acute treatment of inpatients with psychotic symptoms using Acceptance and Commitment Therapy: pilot results. Behav Res Ther 44:415–437, 2006

Gaudiano BA, Miller IW, Herbert JD: The treatment of psychotic major depression: is there a role for adjunctive psychotherapy? Psychother Psychosom 76:271–277, 2007

Johnson J, Horwath E, Weissman MM: The validity of major depression with psychotic features based on a community sample. Arch Gen Psychiatry 48:1075–1081, 1991

Kantrowitz JT, Tampi RR: Risk of psychosis exacerbation by tricyclic antidepressants in unipolar major depressive disorder with psychotic features. J Affect Disord 106:279–284, 2008

Kho KH, Van Vreeswijk MF, Simpson S, et al: A meta-analysis of electroconvulsive therapy efficacy in depression. J ECT 19:139–147, 2003

Kroessler D: Relative efficacy rates for therapies of delusional depression. Convuls Ther 1:173–182, 1985

Meyers BS, Klimstra SA, Gabriele M, et al: Continuation treatment of delusional depression in older adults. Am J Geriatr Psychiatry 9:415–422, 2001

Meyers BS, Flint AJ, Rothschild AJ, et al; for the STOP-PD Study Group: The efficacy of combination pharmacotherapy compared to atypical antipsychotic monotherapy for major depression with psychotic features (Symposium 68C), in Syllabus and Proceedings Summary, American Psychiatric Association Annual Meeting, Washington, DC, May 3–8, 2008. Washington, DC, American Psychiatric Association, 2008, p 179

Müller-Siecheneder F, Müller MJ, Hiller A, et al: Risperidone versus haloperidol and amitriptyline in the treatment of patients with a combined psychotic and depressive syndrome. J Clin Psychopharmacol 18:111–120, 1998

Mulsant BH, Haskett RF, Prudic J, et al: Low use of neuroleptic drugs in the treatment of psychotic major depression. Am J Psychiatry 154:559–561, 1997

Mulsant BH, Sweet RA, Rosen J, et al: A randomized double-blind comparison of nortriptyline plus perphenazine vs. nortriptyline plus placebo in the treatment of psychotic depression in late life. J Clin Psychiatry 62:597–604, 2001

Murphy E: The prognosis of depression in old age. Br J Psychiatry 142:111–119, 1983

Narayan M, Meckler L, Nelson JC: Fluoxetine-induced delusions in psychotic depression (letter). J Clin Psychiatry 56:329, 1995

Nelson JC, Mazure CM: Lithium augmentation in psychotic depression refractory to combined drug treatment. Am J Psychiatry 143:363–366, 1986

Nelson JC, Bowers MB, Sweeney DR: Exacerbation of psychosis by tricyclic antidepressants in delusional depression. Am J Psychiatry 136:574–576, 1979

Olfson M, Marcus S, Sackeim HA, et al: Use of ECT for the inpatient treatment of recurrent major depression. Am J Psychiatry 155:2–29, 1998

Pande AC, Grunhaus LJ, Haskett RF, et al: Electroconvulsive therapy in delusional and non-delusional depressive disorder. J Affect Disord 19:215–219, 1990

Parker G, Roy K, Hadzi-Pavlovic D, et al: Psychotic (delusional) depression: a meta-analysis of physical treatments. J Affect Disord 24:17–24, 1992

Penney JF, Dinwiddie SH, Zorumski CF, et al: Concurrent and close temporal administration of lithium and ECT. Convuls Ther 6:139–145, 1990

Petrides G, Fink M, Husain MM, et al: ECT remission rates in psychotic versus nonpsychotic depressed patients: a report from CORE. J ECT 17:244–253, 2001

Price LH, Conwell Y, Nelson JC: Lithium augmentation of combined neuroleptic-tricyclic treatment in delusional depression. Am J Psychiatry 140:318–322, 1983

Prudic J, Peyser S, Sackeim HA: Subjective memory complaints: a review of patient self-assessment of memory after electroconvulsive therapy. J ECT 16:121–132, 2000

Prudic J, Olfson M, Marchus SC, et al: Effectiveness of electroconvulsive therapy in community settings. Biol Psychiatry 55:301–312, 2004

Rothschild AJ: Management of psychotic, treatment resistant depression. Psychiatr Clin North Am 19:237–252, 1996

Rothschild AJ, Duval SE: How long should patients with psychotic depression stay on the antipsychotic medication? J Clin Psychiatry 64:390–396, 2003

Rothschild AJ, Phillips KA: Selective serotonin reuptake inhibitors and delusional depression. Am J Psychiatry 156:977–978, 1999

Rothschild AJ, Samson JA, Bessette MP, et al: Efficacy of combination fluoxetine and perphenazine in the treatment of psychotic depression. J Clin Psychiatry 54:338–342, 1993

Rothschild AJ, Williamson DJ, Tohen MF, et al: A double-blind, randomized study of olanzapine and olanzapine/fluoxetine combination for major depression with psychotic features. J Clin Psychopharmacol 24:365–373, 2004

Sachs GS, Printz DJ, Kahn DA, et al: The Expert Consensus Guideline Series: medication treatment of bipolar disorder 2000. Postgrad Med (spec no):1–104, 2000

Sackeim HA, Prudic J, Devanand DP, et al: The impact of medication resistance and continuation pharmacotherapy on relapse following response to electroconvulsive therapy in major depression. J Clin Psychopharmacol 10:96–104, 1990

Sackeim HA, Prudic J, Devanand DP, et al: Effects of stimulus intensity and electrode placement on the efficacy and cognitive effects of electroconvulsive therapy. N Engl J Med 328:839–846, 1993

Sackeim HA, Devanand DP, Nobler MS: Electroconvulsive therapy, in Psychopharmacology: The Fourth Generation of Progress. Edited by Bloom F, Kupfer D. New York, Raven, 1995, pp 1123–1142

Sackeim HA, Haskett RF, Mulsant BH, et al: Continuation pharmacotherapy in the prevention of relapse following electroconvulsive therapy: a randomized controlled trial. JAMA 285:1299–1307, 2001

Simpson GM, El Sheshai A, Rady A, et al: Sertraline as a monotherapy in the treatment of psychotic and nonpsychotic depression. J Clin Psychiatry 64:959–965, 2003

Smith E, Rothschild AJ, Heo M, et al; for the Study of Pharmacotherapy of Psychotic Depression (STOP-PD) Collaborative Study Group: Weight gain during olanzapine treatment for psychotic depression: effects of dose and age. Int Clin Psychopharmacol 23:130–137, 2008

Spiker DG, Stein J, Rich CL: Delusional depression and electroconvulsive therapy: one year later. Convuls Ther 1:167–172, 1985a

Spiker DG, Weiss JC, Dealy RS, et al: The pharmacological treatment of delusional depression. Am J Psychiatry 142:430–436, 1985b

Strotskopf C, Horn SD: Predicting length of stay for patients with psychosis. Health Serv Res 26:743–766, 1992

Thompson JW, Weiner RD, Myers CP: Use of ECT in the United States in 1975, 1980, and 1986. Am J Psychiatry 151:1657–1661, 1994

Vythilingam M, Chen J, Bremner JD, et al: Psychotic depression and mortality. Am J Psychiatry 160:574–576, 2003

Weiner RD, Whanger AD, Erwin CW, et al: Prolonged confusional state and EEG seizure activity following concurrent ECT and lithium use. Am J Psychiatry 137:1452–1453, 1980

Wijkstra J, Lijmer J, Balk FJ, et al: Pharmacological treatment for unipolar psychotic depression. Br J Psychiatry 188:410–415, 2006

Wijkstra JJ, Burger D, van den Broek WW, et al: Pharmacological treatment of psychotic depression: a randomized, double-blind study comparing imipramine, venlafaxine, and venlafaxine plus quetiapine (NR5-102), in 2008 New Research Program and Abstracts, American Psychiatric Association 161st Annual Meeting, Washington, DC, May 3–8, 2008. Washington, DC, American Psychiatric Association, 2008, p 259

Wilson KG, Kraitberg NJ, Brown JH, et al: Electroconvulsive therapy in the treatment of depression: the impact on length of stay. Compr Psychiatry 32:345–354, 1991

Zanardi R, Franchini L, Gasperini M, et al: Double-blind controlled trial of sertraline versus paroxetine in the treatment of delusional depression. Am J Psychiatry 153:1631–1633, 1996

Zanardi R, Franchini L, Gasperini M, et al: Faster onset of action of fluvoxamine in combination with pindolol in the treatment of delusional depression: a controlled study. J Clin Psychopharmacol 18:441–446, 1998

Zanardi R, Franchini L, Serritti A, et al: Venlafaxine versus fluvoxamine in the treatment of delusional depression: a pilot double-blind controlled study. J Clin Psychiatry 61:26–29, 2000

Recommended Reading

Andreescu C, Mulsant BH, Peasley-Micklus C, et al; for the STOP-PD Study Group: Persisting low use of antipsychotics in the treatment of major depressive disorder with psychotic features. J Clin Psychiatry 68:194–200, 2007

Gaudiano BA, Miller IW, Herbert JD: The treatment of psychotic major depression: is there a role for adjunctive psychotherapy? Psychother Psychosom 76:271–277, 2007

Prudic J, Olfson M, Marchus SC, et al: Effectiveness of electroconvulsive therapy in community settings. Biol Psychiatry 55:301–312, 2004

Rothschild AJ, Williamson DJ, Tohen MF, et al: A double-blind, randomized study of olanzapine and olanzapine/fluoxetine combination for major depression with psychotic features. J Clin Psychopharmacol 24:365–373, 2004

Sackeim HA, Haskett RF, Mulsant BH, et al: Continuation pharmacotherapy in the prevention of relapse following electroconvulsive therapy: a randomized controlled trial. JAMA 285:1299–1307, 2001

7

Course and Cognition

Short-Term Course

When a patient or family member asks how much time is needed to recover from an episode of psychotic depression, a clinician usually cannot give a precise answer. Some patients respond quickly to treatment, with fast resolution of depressive and psychotic symptoms, whereas other patients may have only partial improvement in symptoms, with a significant period of time elapsing until full recovery. First-episode patients with psychotic depression are more likely to recover symptomatically and functionally (81% recovered) by 6 months than are patients with other psychotic disorders (range of recovery= 36%–70%) (Tohen et al. 2000). In one study, although patients with psychotic depression had had greater psychosocial impairment in the 5 years prior to study entry, after the first 6 months of treatment, they were as likely to recover over the next 18 months as were patients with nonpsychotic depression (Coryell et al. 1987). This study also demonstrated that early response to treatment is more predictive of the later course for patients with psychotic depression than for patients with nonpsychotic depression (Coryell et al. 1987).

If a person has had episodes of psychotic depression in the past, then the amount of time required for the person to recover in the past is often a good predictor of the amount of time needed to recover from the current episode. In general, patients with psychotic depression take longer to recover and return to their baseline level of functioning than do patients with nonpsychotic depression. Compared with patients with nonpsychotic depression, patients with psychotic depression exhibit increased use of services, greater disability, and poorer clinical course at short-term follow-up (Coryell et al. 1986; Rothschild et al. 1993) (see Table 7–1). Patients with psychotic depression have higher rates of suicide and suicide attempts than do patients with nonpsychotic depression (see Chapter 10, "Special Populations and Issues").

Psychotic depression tends to be a more recurrent illness than nonpsychotic depression. A study examining rehospitalization after first admission found that patients with psychotic depression were readmitted sooner (45% less time out of hospital) than patients with nonpsychotic depression (Kessing 2003). Patients with psychotic depression also exhibit more frequent relapses or recurrences than do patients with nonpsychotic depression (Aronson et al. 1987, 1988a, 1988b; Baldwin and Jolley 1986; Coryell et al. 1996; Helms and Smith 1983; E. Lykouras et al. 1986; Murphy 1983; J.C. Nelson and Bowers 1978; Robinson and Spiker 1985; Rothschild and Schatzberg 1993; Spiker et al. 1985), although not all studies are in agreement (Coryell et al. 1987; L. Lykouras et al. 1994).

Long-Term Course

Once a patient has had an episode of psychotic depression, the risk of having psychotic features during future episodes of depression is substantial (see Table 7–2). Recurrence of psychotic features has been most

Table 7–1. Psychotic depression: short-term course

First episode: 81% recovered by 6 months[a]
Early response to treatment predicts later course
Compared with nonpsychotic depression:
↑ Use of services
↑ Disability
↑ Rates of suicide and suicide attempts

[a]Tohen et al. 2000.

extensively examined in an 8-year follow-up study of 424 patients with major depression (Coryell et al. 1994). Of the three subtypes of major depression studied, the psychotic subtype was more consistent across episodes than the endogenous or psychomotorically disturbed subtypes. Patients who had been diagnosed with psychotic depression at intake had a 4- to 15-fold higher risk of being psychotic during subsequent episodes of depression. One study found a striking 86.5% relapse rate into depression over 32 months, with almost all relapses including psychotic features (Aronson et al. 1988a) and the majority of relapses (82.5%) occurring within the first year following discharge. Another study found that recurrence of psychosis, judged either retrospectively or prospectively, had occurred or did eventually occur in 92% of patients (Helms and Smith 1983). However, compared with patients with schizophrenia, patients with psychotic depression were less likely to have delusional symptoms on three separate follow-ups (Harrow et al. 1995).

The proportion of the population that has recurrent psychotic depression versus single episodes is not fully known, although some studies suggest that older patients may have a greater propensity for relapse than younger patients. One study found that patients with late-life psychotic depression were more likely to relapse than were patients with late-life nonpsychotic depression, especially when receiving mainte-

Table 7–2. Psychotic depression: long-term course

Compared with nonpsychotic depression:
↑ Rate of psychosis in future episodes
↑ Rate of rehospitalization[a]
↑ Relapses and recurrences[a]
↑ Residual social and occupational impairment
↑ Risk of suicide
↑ Mortality from medical causes

[a]Particularly in first 12 months after hospitalization.

nance antidepressant monotherapy only (Flint and Rifat 1998). In the most extensively studied cohort to date, Coryell and coworkers (1996) found that individuals with psychotic depression relapsed approximately three times faster than patients with nonpsychotic depression.

Several studies have demonstrated residual social and occupational impairment in patients with psychotic depression despite improvement in psychotic and depressive symptoms at 1-year (Rothschild et al. 1993), 5-year (Coryell et al. 1990), and 10-year (Coryell et al. 1996) follow-ups. However, a 40-year follow-up study found no consistent trends distinguishing patients with psychotic depression from patients with nonpsychotic depression on marital, occupational, residential, or symptomatic outcome ratings (Coryell and Tsuang 1982). The social and occupational impairment has been hypothesized to be secondary to subtle cognitive deficits associated with the higher cortisol levels frequently observed in patients with psychotic depression (Rothschild et al. 1993; Schatzberg and Rothschild 1988; see also Chapter 4, "Biology").

Mortality Rates

Compared with patients with nonpsychotic depression, patients with psychotic depression have higher rates of mortality independent of the higher risk for suicide (for discussion of suicide, see Chapter 10, "Special Populations and Issues"). In a 15-year follow-up of patients with psychotic or nonpsychotic depression (Vythilingam et al. 2003), the mortality rate for subjects with psychotic depression was significantly greater (41%) than that for patients with a diagnosis of nonpsychotic depression (20%). The higher mortality among patients with psychotic depression was not explained by a higher number of suicides, because most of the deaths (88%) were from medical causes.

The increased mortality rates observed in psychotic depression may be related to the chronic dysregulation of the hypothalamic-pituitary-adrenal (HPA) axis that frequently occurs in patients with psychotic depression (see Chapter 4, "Biology"). In one follow-up study, Coryell and colleagues (2008) reported that patients with psychotic depression who died from cardiovascular disease had had significantly higher post-dexamethasone cortisol concentrations than had patients with psychotic depression who did not die of cardiovascular disease. HPA axis hyperactivity also predicted, to a limited extent, death from suicide (Coryell et al. 2008).

Cognitive Disturbances

Complicating the course of psychotic depression (in addition to the psychotic symptoms) are patients' deficits in cognition (see Table 7–3). Patients with psychotic depression typically experience a decrease in speed of mental processing and attention problems with easy distractibility. Every study of psychotic depression that has assessed speed of mental processing using the Trail Making Test or the Digit Symbol subtest of the Wechsler Adult Intelligence Scale—Revised has observed slower mental processing by patients with psychotic depression than by patients with nonpsychotic depression (Jeste et al. 1996; Schatzberg et al. 2000; Simpson et al. 1999). In studies of attentional functioning, impairment in patients with psychotic depression has been observed on measures of immediate auditory attention (Digit Span: Jeste et al. 1996;

Table 7–3. Cognitive disturbances in patients with psychotic depression

Compared with nonpsychotic depression:
↓ Executive functioning
↓ Speed of mental processing
↓ Attention (with easy distractibility)
↓ Verbal memory
↓ Psychomotor speed

Simpson et al. 1999), response inhibition (Stroop Color-Word Test: Schatzberg et al. 2000), and sustained attention and vigilance (Digit Vigilance Test: Jeste et al. 1996; Continuous Performance Test: E.B. Nelson et al. 1998).

Some studies have found that patients with psychotic depression exhibit a pattern of global and diffuse neuropsychological impairment across measures of attention, speed of processing, visual-spatial abilities, learning, memory, and language (Basso and Bornstein 1999). Other studies have found more specific impairment in abstract reasoning and conceptual processing. For example, Kim and colleagues (1999) reported impairment on the Wisconsin Card Sorting Test in a study of geriatric patients with psychotic depression. Similarly, but using a younger sample of patients, Simpson and colleagues (1999) reported greater deficits on the Wisconsin Card Sorting Test in patients with psychotic depression than in patients with nonpsychotic depression.

In three studies (Hill et al. 2004; Jeste et al. 1996; E.B. Nelson et al. 1998), patients with psychotic depression were compared with patients with schizophrenia and patients with nonpsychotic depression. The consistent observation was that the neuropsychological profile of psychotic depression is more similar to that of schizophrenia than to that of nonpsychotic depression. Fleming and colleagues (2004) performed a meta-analysis of five neuropsychological studies of patients with psychotic depression and reported that the greatest cognitive deficits (compared to patients with nonpsychotic depression) were in verbal memory, executive functioning, and psychomotor speed.

A particularly instructive study is that of Hill and colleagues (2004), who compared antipsychotic-naive, first-episode young adults with psychotic depression with antipsychotic-naive, first-episode patients with schizophrenia, antipsychotic-naive patients with nonpsychotic unipolar depression (not first episode), and healthy control subjects. According to the authors, the significant similarities between the neuropsychological profile of the group with schizophrenia and the profile of the group with psychotic depression suggest that similar brain systems may be affected in both of these disorders. In contrast, the cognitive profile for patients with nonpsychotic depression differed dramatically from that for patients with psychotic depression and was more consistent with the cognitive profile for the healthy comparison subjects. The level of performance on neuropsychological testing was generally lower in patients with psychotic depression than in patients with nonpsychotic depression, and those two groups demonstrated statistically significant differences in visual-spatial perception (Hill et al. 2004).

The neuropsychological deficits associated with psychotic depression that were observed in a study by Hill and colleagues (2004) were not attributable to previous exposure to antipsychotic medication or chronic disease effects. Thus, psychosis appears to be associated with a common profile of diffuse neurocognitive dysfunction, regardless of whether it occurs in the context of schizophrenia or depression. Additional studies are needed to assess whether the cognitive impairment persists over the long term; however, long-term studies of the social and occupational functioning of patients with psychotic depression (Coryell et al. 1990, 1996; Rothschild et al. 1993) suggest that cognitive impairment might persist. Whether there are differences in cognitive functioning associated with early-onset versus late-onset psychotic depression and whether it is possible to identify etiological factors underlying the neuropsychological deficits observed in patients with psychotic depression are questions for future research.

Key Clinical Points

- First-episode patients with psychotic depression are more likely to recover symptomatically and functionally by 6 months than are patients with other psychotic disorders.
- Patients with psychotic depression have higher rates of suicide, suicide attempts, and mortality due to medical causes than do patients with nonpsychotic depression.
- Patients with psychotic depression have higher rates of relapse, recurrence, and rehospitalization than do patients with nonpsychotic depression.
- Older patients may have a greater propensity for relapse than younger patients.
- Patients with psychotic depression have more cognitive problems, as measured by neuropsychological testing, than do patients with nonpsychotic depression.

References

Aronson TA, Shukla S, Hoff A: Continuation therapy after ECT for delusional depression: a naturalistic study of prophylactic treatments and relapse. Convuls Ther 3:251–259, 1987

Aronson TA, Shukla S, Gujavarty K, et al: Relapse in delusional depression: a retrospective study of the course of treatment. Compr Psychiatry 29:12–21, 1988a

Aronson TA, Shukla S, Hoff A, et al: Proposed delusional depression subtypes: preliminary evidence from a retrospective study of phenomenology and treatment course. J Affect Disord 14:69–74, 1988b

Baldwin RC, Jolley DJ: The prognosis of depression in old age. Br J Psychiatry 149:574–583, 1986

Basso MR, Bornstein RA: Neuropsychological deficits in psychotic versus non-psychotic unipolar depression. Neuropsychology 13:69–75, 1999
Coryell W, Tsuang MT: Primary unipolar depression and the prognostic importance of delusions. Arch Gen Psychiatry 39:1181–1184, 1982
Coryell W, Zimmerman M, Pfohl B: Outcome at discharge and six months in major depression: the significance of psychotic features. J Nerv Ment Dis 174:92–96, 1986
Coryell W, Endicott J, Keller M: The importance of psychotic features to major depression: course and outcome during a 2-year follow-up. Acta Psychiatr Scand 75:78–85, 1987
Coryell W, Keller M, Lavori P, et al: Affective syndromes, psychotic features and prognosis, I: depression. Arch Gen Psychiatry 47:651–657, 1990
Coryell W, Winokur G, Shea T, et al: The long-term stability of depressive subtypes. Am J Psychiatry 151:199–204, 1994
Coryell W, Leon A, Winokur G, et al: The importance of psychotic features to long term course in depressive disorders. Am J Psychiatry 153:483–489, 1996
Coryell W, Fiedorowicz J, Zimmerman M, et al: HPA-axis hyperactivity and mortality in psychotic depressive disorder: preliminary findings. Psychoneuroendocrinology 3:654–658, 2008
Fleming SK, Blasey C, Schatzberg AF: Neuropsychological correlates of psychotic features in major depressive disorders: a review and meta-analysis. J Psychiatr Res 38:27–35, 2004
Flint AJ, Rifat SL: Two-year outcome of psychotic depression in late life. Am J Psychiatry 155:178–183, 1998
Harrow M, MacDonald AW III, Sands JR, et al: Vulnerability to delusions over time in schizophrenia and affective disorders. Schizophr Bull 21:95–109, 1995
Helms PM, Smith RE: Recurrent psychotic depression: evidence of diagnostic stability. J Affect Disord 5:51–54, 1983
Hill SK, Keshavan MS, Thase ME, et al: Neuropsychological dysfunction in antipsychotic-naive first-episode unipolar psychotic depression. Am J Psychiatry 161:996–1003, 2004
Jeste DV, Heaton SC, Paulsen JS, et al: Clinical and neuropsychological comparison of psychotic depression with nonpsychotic depression and schizophrenia. Am J Psychiatry 153:490–496, 1996

Kessing LV: Subtypes of depressive episodes according to ICD-10: prediction of risk of relapse and suicide. Psychopathology 36:285–291, 2003

Kim DK, Kim BL, Sohn SE, et al: Candidate neuroanatomic substrates of psychosis in old-aged depression. Prog Neuropsychopharmacol Biol Psychiatry 23:793–807, 1999

Lykouras E, Malliaras D, Christodoulou GN, et al: Delusional depression: phenomenology and response to treatment: a prospective study. Acta Psychiatr Scand 73:324–329, 1986

Lykouras L, Christodoulou GN, Malliaras D, et al: The prognostic importance of delusions in depression: a 6-year prospective follow-up study. J Affect Disord 32:233–238, 1994

Murphy E: The prognosis of depression in old age. Br J Psychiatry 142:111–119, 1983

Nelson EB, Sax KW, Strakowski SM: Attentional performance in patients with psychotic and nonpsychotic major depression and schizophrenia. Am J Psychiatry 155:137–139, 1998

Nelson JC, Bowers MB: Delusional versus unipolar depression: description and drug response. Arch Gen Psychiatry 35:1321–1328, 1978

Robinson DG, Spiker DG: Delusional depression: a one year follow-up. J Affect Disord 9:79–83, 1985

Rothschild AJ, Schatzberg AF: Psychotic depression: a newly recognized subtype. Clin Neurosci 1:75–80, 1993

Rothschild AJ, Samson JA, Bond TC, et al: Hypothalamic-pituitary-adrenal axis activity and one-year outcome in depression. Biol Psychiatry 34:392–400, 1993

Schatzberg AF, Rothschild AJ: The roles of glucocorticoid and dopaminergic systems in delusional (psychotic) depression. Ann N Y Acad Sci 537:462–471, 1988

Schatzberg AF, Posener JA, DeBattista C, et al: Neuropsychological deficits in psychotic versus nonpsychotic major depression and no mental illness. Am J Psychiatry 157:1095–1100, 2000

Simpson S, Baldwin RC, Jackson A, et al: The differentiation of DSM-III-R psychotic depression in later life from nonpsychotic depression: comparisons of brain changes measured by multispectral analysis of magnetic resonance brain images, neuropsychological findings, and clinical features. Biol Psychiatry 45:193–204, 1999

Spiker DG, Stein J, Rich CL: Delusional depression and electroconvulsive therapy: one year later. Convuls Ther 1:167–172, 1985

Tohen M, Strakowski SM, Zarate C Jr, et al: The McLean-Harvard first-episode project: 6-month symptomatic and functional outcome in affective and nonaffective psychosis. Biol Psychiatry 48:467–476, 2000

Vythilingam M, Chen J, Bremner JD, et al: Psychotic depression and mortality. Am J Psychiatry 160:574–576, 2003

Recommended Reading

Coryell W, Winokur G, Shea T, et al: The long-term stability of depressive subtypes. Am J Psychiatry 151:199–204, 1994

Coryell W, Leon A, Winokur G, et al: The importance of psychotic features to long term course in depressive disorders. Am J Psychiatry 153:483–489, 1996

Hill SK, Keshavan MS, Thase ME, et al: Neuropsychological dysfunction in antipsychotic-naive first-episode unipolar psychotic depression. Am J Psychiatry 161:996–1003, 2004

Vythilingam M, Chen J, Bremner JD, et al: Psychotic depression and mortality. Am J Psychiatry 160:574–576, 2003

8

Treatment Settings

The primary factors to consider when determining the appropriate level of care for a patient with psychotic depression are the patient's potential for self-harm, potential to harm others, and ability to care for himself or herself. Because significant morbidity and mortality occur in patients with psychotic depression from both medical causes (Vythilingam et al. 2003) and suicide (see Chapter 10, "Special Populations and Issues"), the placement of these patients in appropriate settings is critical. Table 8–1 lists various settings for patients with psychotic depression.

Hospitalization

Many individuals with psychotic depression require hospitalization. Both inpatients and outpatients were accepted as participants in the National Institute of Mental Health's Study of the Pharmacotherapy of Psychotic Depression; in this study, 69% of the 259 subjects with psy-

Table 8–1. Levels of care for patients with psychotic depression

Hospitalization
Partial hospitalization
Intensive day treatment
Intensive outpatient treatment
Outpatient treatment

chotic depression were inpatients (Meyers et al. 2008). Inpatient hospitalization removes the patient from outside stressors, enables closer monitoring of the patient's response to treatment, and allows more aggressive titration of psychotropic medications than can occur in outpatient treatment. Also, if electroconvulsive therapy (ECT) is being given, inpatient hospitalization allows for closer assessment of the patient's response and cognition on a day when he or she is not receiving ECT.

Inpatient milieu treatment is based on the belief that interpersonal and group processes can help promote corrective emotional experiences, promote psychological growth, and help the patient with psychotic depression to rehabilitate. Evidence for the beneficial effects of an inpatient therapeutic milieu for psychotic depression comes, somewhat ironically, from a pharmacologic treatment study (Rothschild et al. 2004). In this study, which is the only double-blind, placebo-controlled study of patients with psychotic depression carried out in an inpatient setting, response rates of the placebo group in the two independent trials were 28% and 31%. Although the so-called placebo group received no active pharmacologic treatment, the response rates for the placebo group most likely reflect the benefits of inpatient hospitalization: removal from a stressful situation, empathic staff rendering individual and group psychotherapy, and psychoeducation of the patients and their families. (For details regarding nursing care of the patient with psychotic depression, see Chapter 9, "Nursing Care.")

In this era of managed care, the inpatient stay of the patient with psychotic depression is likely to be brief, although it is usually longer than that of the patient with nonpsychotic depression. Inpatient hospitalizations of patients with psychotic depression are prolonged because of specific symptoms: severe depression, psychosis, suicidal ideation and behaviors, homicidal ideation (particularly in postpartum psychotic depression), and inability to care for self (see Table 8–2).

No patient, for economic or other reasons, should be released from a secure inpatient setting until the staff members have judged that it is safe for the patient to leave. Unfortunately, the clinician is often faced with discharging the patient before it is clear whether the somatic treatment rendered (medications or ECT) is going to be fully effective. Furthermore, any improvement seen in the patient after admission may be secondary to the nonsomatic treatments rendered.

Before being discharged, the patient needs to be carefully evaluated for the potential risk of suicide (and homicide, if applicable; see section "Postpartum Psychotic Depression" in Chapter 10, "Special Populations and Issues"). In particular, if, prior to admission, the patient made a suicide attempt that was based on a delusional belief, the clinician needs to assess the patient to be sure that the delusions have abated. In my experience, the delusions often get better quickly (sometimes, but not always, in days), whereas the depressive symptoms can take considerably longer to improve (on the order of weeks to months). Some large studies of psychotic depression have reported improvement in some patients within a week (Meyers et al. 2008; Rothschild et al. 2004). However, no study has considered whether any significant improvement occurs in less than a week, which unfortunately is the typical length of stay in many hospitals.

An effective therapeutic alliance, evidence of hope for the future, reliable social supports, and continuity of therapeutic care can permit acutely ill patients with psychotic depression to be discharged while still somewhat symptomatic. Obviously, the posthospital treatment plan is of critical importance. Implementation of the posthospital treat-

Table 8–2. Symptoms of psychotic depression that can prolong hospitalization

Severe depression
Psychotic symptoms
Suicidal ideation and behaviors
Homicidal ideation (more common in postpartum psychotic depression)
Inability to care for self

ment plan should occur immediately after discharge, which is a time of increased risk. The patient with psychotic depression is often returning to a life with the same stressors that were present prior to the hospitalization and is in the middle of a treatment regimen whose effectiveness cannot yet be ascertained. Therefore, close follow-up beginning immediately upon discharge is important.

Involuntary Commitment

At times, an acutely ill patient with psychotic depression may pose a danger to self or others and may require hospitalization on an involuntary basis. Clinicians may find themselves in very difficult situations, such as being responsible for an involuntarily committed patient but having no authority to treat the patient (because of the patient's right to refuse medication except in an emergency). Furthermore, the somatic treatment modalities used to treat psychotic depression (see Chapter 6, "Treatment") are limited with an involuntary patient. Antidepressants cannot be given by injection, and a court is unlikely to order ECT against a patient's will. Thus, the clinician's only somatic treatment option for an involuntary patient is injectable antipsychotic medication. Although antipsychotic monotherapy is not the most effective treatment for psychotic depression (see Chapter 6, "Treatment"), the use of antipsychotics may allow sufficient improvement that the patient later accepts either an antidepressant–antipsychotic combination or ECT.

The clinician may also have concerns about his or her potential liability for a patient's dangerousness after discharge. Clinicians should render care using their best clinical judgments, keeping in mind that predictive accuracy of a patient's dangerousness is limited. The less restrictive settings discussed in the remainder of this chapter may offer appropriate options for the recently discharged patient with psychotic depression.

Outpatient Commitment

Outpatient commitment—sometimes called *assisted outpatient treatment*—is a court order combined with outpatient treatment for individuals with severe psychiatric disorders. This type of care is available in 42 states in the United States. Outpatient commitment may have a role in decreasing rates of hospitalization in patients with psychotic depression.

Partial Hospitalization and Intensive Day Treatment

Partial hospitalization and intensive day treatment programs can provide structured activities and social skills training for a patient with psychotic depression who requires almost daily monitoring but who is not at high risk for dangerous behavior. These programs can be used for patients who have recently been discharged from an inpatient unit or can be used initially as an alternative to inpatient hospitalization. Like inpatient units, these programs can allow daily monitoring of patients and the opportunity to closely assess the patients for response to treatment. These settings may also allow more aggressive titration of psychotropic medications than can occur in outpatient treatment. Similarly, for patients receiving ECT, these programs allow for assessment of the patients' response and cognition on a day when they are not receiving ECT. If ECT has been started on the inpatient unit, the partial hospitalization and day treatment programs can be used to continue or complete the course of ECT. The goal is to continue intensive inpatient care in a less restrictive setting or to avoid an inpatient hospitalization. Partial hospitalization and intensive day treatment require a voluntary patient who is motivated to participate in outpatient treatment and has adequate social supports at home in the evening and at night.

Intensive Outpatient Treatment

Intensive outpatient treatment provides a level of care for patients with psychotic depression who require frequent contact for assessment and management. Most patients with psychotic depression who are discharged from an inpatient setting in less than a week require at least this level of care so their response to medications or ECT can be properly assessed. The interventions used in intensive outpatient treatment may include increased frequencies of regular outpatient therapies such as individual psychotherapy, group therapy, couples therapy, family therapy, occupational therapy, and rehabilitation services, as well as easy and immediate access to psychopharmacologic consultation. The goal of intensive outpatient treatment is continued stabilization of the patient to prevent relapse requiring hospitalization.

Outpatient Treatment

The outpatient treatment team plays a critical role in the long-term management of the patient with psychotic depression. As discussed in Chapter 7 ("Course and Cognition"), patients with psychotic depression have high rates of relapse and recurrence, of suicide, and of mortality from medical causes. Thus, an integrated approach that combines psychiatric and medical services in a comprehensive way is best for the long-term management of the patient with psychotic depression.

Outpatient approaches include psychopharmacology and psychosocial treatments such as cognitive-behavioral therapy, individual psychotherapy, couples therapy, family therapy, and group therapy. Ideally, outpatient clinicians should have familiarity with psychotic depression, particularly the challenges in assessing patients who are not always forthcoming about their psychotic symptoms (see Chapter 5, "Diagnosis and Assessment"). The goal of outpatient therapists should be to develop a strong therapeutic alliance with each patient, so that if and when the patient starts to have delusional symptoms again, he or she will feel comfortable confiding in the outpatient treatment team.

If the clinician did not develop a relationship with the family during the patient's inpatient hospitalization, establishing such a relationship should be a goal during outpatient treatment. The clinician must first educate family members about psychotic depression, emphasizing that although it is a treatable illness, there is a significant degree of morbidity and mortality. Education regarding the treatment being rendered and its side effects is also important. Educating the family about the illness may help to reduce guilt. Information about the type and length of treatment and expectations for change will reduce anxiety. As observers of any unusual thoughts or behaviors that the patient may be exhibiting, family members play a key role in helping to recognize a possible relapse or recurrence of psychotic depression.

Key Clinical Points

- A large percentage of patients with psychotic depression require inpatient hospitalization.
- Inpatient hospitalization removes the patient from outside stressors and allows closer monitoring of the patient's response to treatment.
- Inpatient hospitalization of the patient with psychotic depression can be prolonged because of several symptoms: severe depression, psychosis, suicidal ideation and behaviors, homicidal ideation (particularly in postpartum psychotic depression), and inability to care for self.

- Partial hospitalization, intensive day treatment, intensive outpatient treatment, and outpatient treatment play key roles in the rehabilitation of the patient with psychotic depression.
- If the clinician did not develop a relationship with the family during the patient's inpatient hospitalization, this should be a goal during outpatient treatment.

References

Meyers BS, Flint AJ, Rothschild AJ, et al; for the STOP-PD Study Group: The efficacy of combination pharmacotherapy compared to atypical antipsychotic monotherapy for major depression with psychotic features (Symposium 68C), in Syllabus and Proceedings Summary, American Psychiatric Association Annual Meeting, Washington, DC, May 3–8, 2008. Washington, DC, American Psychiatric Association, 2008, p 179

Rothschild AJ, Williamson DJ, Tohen MF, et al: A double-blind, randomized study of olanzapine and olanzapine/fluoxetine combination for major depression with psychotic features. J Clin Psychopharmacol 24:365–373, 2004

Vythilingam M, Chen J, Bremner JD, et al: Psychotic depression and mortality. Am J Psychiatry 160:574–576, 2003

Recommended Reading

Joska JA, Stein DJ: Mood disorders, in The American Psychiatric Publishing Textbook of Psychiatry, 5th Edition. Edited by Hales RE, Yudofsky SC, Gabbard GO. Washington, DC, American Psychiatric Publishing, 2008, pp 457–503

9

Nursing Care

Judith Shindul-Rothschild, Ph.D., R.N., C.S.

Patients with psychotic depression are likely to differ from other hospitalized psychiatric patients in the degree to which they require intensive nursing care. Pervasive delusional ideation can immobilize patients to the point that they neglect all self-care activities. Nursing interventions for the patient with psychotic depression include risk assessment and management of basic health care needs; management of medical illnesses and somatic complaints; assessment of efficacy of medications and side effects; ensuring patient adherence to medication and obtaining informed consent for electroconvulsive therapy (ECT); car-

Judith Shindul-Rothschild, Ph.D., R.N., C.S., is Associate Professor and Chair of the Community and Psychiatric Mental Health Nursing Department of the William F. Connell School of Nursing at Boston College in Chestnut Hill, Massachusetts.

ing for patients before and after ECT; assessing women for postpartum psychotic depression; and case management.

Priority Nursing Interventions

Risk Assessment

Nursing staff are responsible for assessing each patient's suicidal ideation and potential for violence, obtaining details about past suicide attempts, and assessing nonverbal cues that may indicate delusions or hallucinations. Nursing assessment and management of patients' safety rely on both environmental safeguards and development of a therapeutic alliance (see Table 9–1).

Decisions about the amount of observation required for each patient are based on the collective judgment of the treatment team; however, nursing staff can, and often do, impose greater restrictions based on their assessment of a patient's impulsivity. Close communication with all members of the treatment team, especially regarding details about past suicide attempts and nonverbal cues that may suggest the patient is responding to internal stimulation, is key in assisting the nursing staff to appropriately assess the patient's level of risk. Standardized suicide assessment tools completed by nursing staff and the psychiatrist on admission, periodically during hospitalization and immediately prior to discharge, can ensure that crucial information is elicited and documented in the medical record about the patient's risk for self-harm (Sullivan et al. 2005).

Collateral information can be very beneficial in risk assessment, especially when the patient may be severely withdrawn and noncommunicative (see Table 9–2). When family and friends visit the patient, nursing staff can inquire about their impressions and concerns. If the patient is transferred from a long-term-care facility, conferring with nursing colleagues about the patient's usual routines, behavior prior to decompensation, and history of self-harm can assist the treatment team in determining the level of observation appropriate at admission.

Table 9–1. Nursing risk assessment of patients with psychotic depression

Develop therapeutic alliance
Assess suicidal ideation
Assess potential for violence
Obtain details about past suicide attempts
Assess nonverbal cues that may indicate delusions or hallucinations

Risk assessment includes frequent therapeutic communication with the patient. A thorough risk assessment is best achieved when the patient is an active participant. However, patients with psychotic depression may be secretive about suicidal intent triggered by delusions or auditory hallucinations, and eliciting information from the patient may be difficult. If the patient with psychotic depression is communicative and oriented, the goal is for nurses and the patient to mutually devise a plan that can best maintain the patient's safety (Buchanan-Barker and Barker 2005). The safety plan would include recognizing nonverbal cues that the patient is unsafe (e.g., pacing or withdrawing to his or her room), identifying triggers to suicidal ideation (e.g., anniversary reaction to the death of a loved one), and helping the patient to develop coping strategies to use when feeling suicidal (e.g., talking to staff or family) (see Table 9–3).

Risk Management

Psychiatric units are designed to minimize the likelihood that patients will commit acts of self-harm. On admission, nursing staff should conduct a thorough examination of the patient's belongings and remove any items that may pose a safety risk. This initial contact with the patient must be conducted with great care and respect for the patient's dignity. Nursing staff typically recommend either one-to-one observation for acutely suicidal patients (the patient always is within arm's length of the

Table 9–2. Tools for nursing risk assessment of patients with psychotic depression

Administer standardized assessment tools
Obtain information from family and friends visiting patient
Confer with nursing colleagues from referring institution
Involve patient as active participant

nurse), close observation (the patient is always within vision of members of the nursing staff), or frequent checks (5–30 minutes apart) by members of the nursing staff. Patients under close observation are restricted to open areas or an area in front of the nursing station, where they are visually observed by members of the nursing staff.

Risk management involves more than ensuring that the environment is safe and the patient is being closely observed. The therapeutic alliance between the nursing staff and patients is essential in minimizing patients' impulses to act on their thoughts to commit self-harm. Although the patient with psychotic depression may appear indifferent to the nursing staff, nursing research indicates that most patients who are hospitalized wish that nursing staff spent more time with them (Sun et al. 2006).

By providing patients with unconditional positive regard and instilling hope for recovery, the nursing staff begin the process of developing an alliance with patients (Koehn and Cutcliffe 2007). Individual interactions in which the nursing staff elicit information and treatment preferences from patients reinforce the commitment of the nursing staff to empower the patients to direct their care as much as possible (Shattell et al. 2006). The therapeutic value of psychiatric nursing practice derives from the presence of the nursing staff, prompt attention to the patients' needs, and responding to the patients' needs with compassion, even with the most mundane activities (Schröder et al. 2006).

Table 9–3. Nursing safety plan for patients with psychotic depression

Recognize nonverbal cues that the patient is unsafe
Identify triggers of suicidal ideation
Help patient develop coping strategies to use when feeling suicidal

Nursing Management of Medical Illnesses and Somatic Complaints

Medical Comorbidities

Individuals with psychotic depression commonly neglect their routine medical care. Women may have neglected routine mammograms, gynecological examinations, or postpartum follow-up examinations. Similarly, men may not have had recent medical examinations or screening for chronic health conditions. One of the challenges of providing nursing care to patients with psychotic depression is the management of medical or somatic conditions (see Table 9–4). Coordination between the psychiatric treatment team and the primary care or long-term-care provider's recommendations for treatment is a key role of the nursing staff. Hospitalization provides an ideal opportunity to schedule patient referrals to multiple health care providers, such as specialists in internal medicine, dentistry, podiatry, or gynecology, for assessment and treatment of medical and somatic symptoms.

One of the factors potentially complicating medical treatment is that the patient may not be capable of consent because of his or her mental status. Emergency guardianship should be sought when the patient's medical status is in jeopardy and the patient is unwilling or unable to provide consent. Clear criteria need to be negotiated between the psychiatrist, nursing staff, and medical staff about the conditions under which emergency guardianship will be sought.

Table 9–4. Nursing management of medical illnesses and somatic complaints

Monitor vital signs
Monitor fluid input and output
Obtain appropriate consultations
Be mindful that somatic complaints could be delusional
Develop behavioral plan for patient participation in the treatment activities of the inpatient setting despite physical symptoms

A patient with psychotic depression may refuse to drink fluids even under supervision. Thus, monitoring of fluid intake and output is very important. To avoid a medical crisis, the treatment team should anticipate, with the guardian, those conditions in which emergency medical care will be provided if the patient continues to resist or refuse care. The nursing treatment plan would also document the measurable criteria, including potassium level, vital signs, weight, and so forth, that would warrant emergency intravenous fluids.

Patients with psychotic depression commonly have somatic complaints, which often include expressions of pain. Ascertaining the etiology of the pain and whether it is associated with delusions can be very challenging for the nursing staff. Headache, stomachache, and bone and back pain should be systematically evaluated by primary care and medical specialists. The treatment team should establish a plan to manage somatic complaints that is consistent for all nursing staff members on all shifts and all prescribing practitioners. For patients who have been prescribed narcotics to treat pain, consultation with a pain specialist in nursing may be warranted. Nursing pain specialists are helpful in assisting all members of the nursing staff to understand the rationale behind the treatment regimen and can offer adjuncts to treatment in addition to analgesic medication.

Cognitive-behavioral therapists can also consult with the nursing staff about therapeutic interventions. For example, if a patient's participation in the treatment activities of the inpatient setting is consistently hampered by somatic complaints (e.g., "I can't attend group therapy because I have a headache"), the nursing staff can develop a behavioral plan that reinforces the patient's attempts to interact constructively in the inpatient setting.

Nursing Interventions

Most patients with psychotic depression have significant self-care deficits and sleep impairments. Mobilizing the patient with psychotic depression to participate in the most routine activity can be an enormous challenge for members of the nursing staff. How much the patient may be expected to participate in self-care versus how much the nursing staff should assist the patient with routine hygiene, bathing, and dressing is a frequent topic of debate in treatment team meetings.

Although patients who are severely preoccupied with their delusions or who are profoundly impaired will require a high intensity of basic nursing care, behavioral programs are appropriate for patients who are not grossly impaired by psychotic thinking. Patients who are incontinent should be placed on a regular toileting schedule and allowed only limited fluids at night. Emaciated patients should be referred for a dietary consultation and given protein shakes as a supplement to meals.

Sleep patterns are often disrupted for patients with psychotic depression. Nursing care plans to promote improved patient sleep should include exercise, exposure to sunlight, eliminating caffeine intake, warm baths, quiet activities such as reading, and a cool room with warm bedding. Sleep hygiene interventions may not be sufficient to normalize sleep. For patients whose sleep-wake cycle has reversed, nursing staff should keep the patient awake an hour longer each night until the pattern has normalized. Melatonin may be prescribed to facilitate sleep, and antipsychotic medication can also be administered in the evening, especially if it has a sedative side effect, to help normalize sleep.

Clinical Exemplars

> On admission, a patient with psychotic depression was very resistant to getting out of his chair to walk. When the nursing staff examined his feet, they found that his toenails were so long they curved around the top of his toe to the underside of his foot. The patient was restricted to his bed until a podiatrist could provide foot and nail care.

> A patient with psychotic depression was reported to be very reclusive and resistant to coming out of her home. The admission referral noted that she believed she was a "witch." The intake nursing assessment noted that the patient was severely emaciated and had long straggly black and gray hair down to her buttocks. She had one discolored tooth visible in the center of her top gum—all other teeth were missing. Nursing staff referred the patient to a dentist and the hospital hairdresser.

Nursing Assessment of Efficacy of Medications and Side Effects

Patients with psychotic depression are likely to be prescribed both antidepressant and antipsychotic medications (see Chapter 6, "Treatment," for further discussion). As outlined in Table 9–5, the nursing assessment of the efficacy of the medications prescribed and their side effects is extremely important.

Frequently, because patients with psychotic depression have somatic complaints, they are also given prescriptions for analgesics and other medications to manage chronic medical conditions. Antianxiety agents, in particular benzodiazepines, may be prescribed to manage sleep or behavioral symptoms. Given the number of classes of pharmacologic agents prescribed to patients with psychotic depression, especially elderly patients, drug–drug interactions are a concern. Hospitalization of the patient provides an ideal opportunity for nurses to confer with all the patient's prescribers to determine whether the medication regimen can be simplified to minimize the likelihood that changes in mental status are a function of drug–drug interactions or side effects.

Table 9–5. Nursing assessment of efficacy of medications and side effects

Assess potential for drug–drug interactions
Identify and document target symptoms
Watch for cumulative anticholinergic side effects
Monitor vital signs (e.g., watch for orthostatic hypotension)
Screen for tardive dyskinesia
Screen for metabolic syndrome

At patient intake, nursing staff should determine the presence and severity of target symptoms that are to be treated with psychotropic medications and document this list in the nursing treatment plan. Nursing staff should note neurovegetative signs and symptoms, such as sleep patterns; activity level; and ability to feed, bathe, and clothe self. Night nurses' notes, which may be overlooked by members of the treatment team, include vital information about a patient's sleep, which is often one of the first target symptoms to improve with treatment. Changes in speech, thought processes, mood, and affect are additional target symptoms that should be noted by all members of the treatment team and recorded daily in the nursing notes.

Anticholinergic side effects can be problematic for the patient with psychotic depression. Reducing polypharmacy and lowering doses of medications with high anticholinergic effects help minimize the potential adverse effects on a patient's mental status. If the patient's mental status continues to deteriorate, or is characterized by confusion, apathy, and unintelligible speech, delirium should be ruled out as a cause. During hospitalization, if the nursing staff observe akathisia or pseudoparkinsonian symptoms, nurses should recommend that the prescriber consider adding an antiparkinsonian or anticholinergic agent. Immobility in combination with anticholinergic side effects can cause constipation, which may lead to impaction. High-fiber diets, stool softeners, and toileting regimens should be routinely included in the nursing care plan.

Orthostatic hypotension is a potential side effect that increases the patient's risk of falls, especially if the patient is elderly or dehydrated. On intake, the nursing assessment should gather information about the patient's risk for falls from referring agencies, the treatment team, and family. Nursing staff should instruct the patient to get out of bed slowly and to maintain adequate levels of hydration. Occupational and physical therapists can be very helpful in providing the patient with walking aids and coaching to improve gait. If the patient is considered at high risk for falling, alarms can be clipped to the patient's clothing to alert the nursing staff if the patient is attempting to walk without assistance.

Routine vital signs can alert the nursing staff to potentially life-threatening side effects of psychotropic medication. Any fever, rash, severe muscle stiffness, severe headache, or abdominal pain warrants immediate referral to the prescribing practitioner by the nursing staff. Nursing staff will request immediate relevant laboratory tests, review all laboratory findings, and alert prescribers about any abnormal findings. Psychotropic medications should not be administered to a patient if the nurse believes that the patient may be exhibiting any symptoms of agranulocytosis, neuroleptic malignant syndrome, cholestatic jaundice, dystonia, priapism, serotonin syndrome, lithium toxicity, respiratory depression, or cardiac arrhythmias.

If the patient exhibits symptoms of tardive dyskinesia, nursing staff should screen the patient, using the Abnormal Involuntary Movement Scale (Guy 1976; see Figure 9–1), at admission or during hospitalization. According to the nursing standard of care, patients who are taking medications that may cause tardive dyskinesia should be screened every 3 months (Varcarolis 2006). For patients taking psychotropic medications that are known to cause significant weight gain, nursing staff should follow guidelines jointly developed by the American Diabetes Association and the American Psychiatric Association for assessment of metabolic syndrome (Straker et al. 2005). When the patient is admitted to the hospital, nursing staff record the patient's weight, blood pressure, and waist circumference. In gathering information on family and personal medical history, nursing staff inquire about diabetes, gestational diabetes, birth weight of children, and hyperlipidemia. If there is evidence of metabolic syndrome or if the nursing staff determine that the patient is at risk for metabolic syndrome, a dietary referral and laboratory tests that include a fasting glucose and fasting lipid profile should be requested.

Medication Adherence and Informed Consent for ECT

Rehospitalization of patients with psychotic symptoms is often precipitated by nonadherence to the medication treatment regimen. Even when patients with psychotic depression are hospitalized, they frequently refuse oral administration of prescribed medication or, when indicated, ECT. It is important for the nursing staff to respond to the patient's complaints or fears with genuine concern. The patient may have delusions that the medication is poison or legitimate worries based on prior experiences. Nursing staff can explore the patient's rationale for refusing medication or ECT and educate the patient about the risks and benefits. If the patient experienced distressing side effects with prior administration of the medication, nursing staff can confer with the prescriber about possible alternatives. Trusted family and friends can be helpful in relaying to the patient their confidence in the medication regimen or the benefit of ECT and remind the patient of prior episodes that were successfully managed with either of the treatments.

Participation in nurse-led medication groups provides the patient who is ambivalent with an additional opportunity to learn more about medication or ECT and to listen to other patients who have experienced similar symptoms and benefited from treatment. Educational films and informational brochures developed by nursing staff or downloaded from trusted Internet sources, such as the National Institute of Mental Health, provide patients and families with additional resources to make

ABNORMAL INVOLUNTARY MOVEMENT SCALE (AIMS)

Patient's Name (Please print)________________ Patient's ID information ________________

Examiner's Name ________________

CURRENT MEDICATIONS AND TOTAL MG/DAY

Medication #1 ________ Total mg/day ________ Medication #2 ________ Total mg/day ________

INSTRUCTIONS: COMPLETE THE EXAMINATION PROCEDURE BEFORE ENTERING THESE RATINGS.

	None, normal	Minimal (may be extreme normal)	Mild	Moderate	Severe
Facial and Oral Movements					
1. **Muscles of Facial Expression** e.g., movements of forehead, eyebrows, periorbital area, cheeks; include frowning, blinking, smiling, grimacing	☐ 0	☐ 1	☐ 2	☐ 3	☐ 4
2. **Lips and Perioral Area** e.g., puckering, pouting, smacking	☐ 0	☐ 1	☐ 2	☐ 3	☐ 4
3. **Jaw** e.g., biting, clenching, chewing, mouth opening, lateral movement	☐ 0	☐ 1	☐ 2	☐ 3	☐ 4
4. **Tongue:** Rate only increases in movement both in and out of mouth, NOT inability to sustain movement.	☐ 0	☐ 1	☐ 2	☐ 3	☐ 4
Extremity Movements					
5. **Upper (arms, wrists, hands, fingers):** Include choreic movements (i.e., rapid, objectively purposeless, irregular, spontaneous); athetoid movements (i.e., slow, irregular, complex, serpentine). DO NOT include tremor (i.e., repetitive, regular, rhythmic).	☐ 0	☐ 1	☐ 2	☐ 3	☐ 4
6. **Lower (legs, knees, ankles, toes)** e.g., lateral knee movement, foot tapping, heel dropping, foot squirming, inversion and eversion of foot	☐ 0	☐ 1	☐ 2	☐ 3	☐ 4

Trunk Movements

7. Neck, shoulders, hips e.g., rocking, twisting, squirming, pelvic gyrations	☐ 0	☐ 1	☐ 2	☐ 3	☐ 4

SCORING

- Score the highest amplitude or frequency in a movement on the 0–4 scale, not the average.
- Score activated movements the same way; do not lower those numbers as was proposed at one time.
- A POSITIVE AIMS EXAMINATION IS A SCORE OF 2 IN TWO OR MORE MOVEMENTS or a SCORE OF 3 OR 4 IN A SINGLE MOVEMENT.
- Do not sum the scores: e.g., a patient who has scores 1 in four movements DOES NOT have a positive AIMS score of 4.

Overall Severity

8. Severity of abnormal movements	☐ 0	☐ 1	☐ 2	☐ 3	☐ 4
9. Incapacitation due to abnormal movements	☐ 0	☐ 1	☐ 2	☐ 3	☐ 4
	No awareness	Aware, no distress	Aware, mild distress	Aware, moderate distress	Aware, severe distress
10. Patient's awareness of abnormal movements (rate only patient's report)	☐ 0	☐ 1	☐ 2	☐ 3	☐ 4

Dental Status

	Yes	No
11. Current problems with teeth and/or dentures?	☐	☐
12. Does patient usually wear dentures?	☐	☐

Comments: ______________________________

Examiner's Signature ______________________ Next Exam Date ______________

Figure 9–1. Abnormal Involuntary Movement Scale.

Source. Reprinted from Guy W: *ECDEU Assessment Manual for Psychopharmacology,* Revised (DHEW Publ No ADM 76-338). Washington, DC, U.S. Department of Health, Education, and Welfare, 1976.

an informed decision about the recommended treatment. Nurses can reassure the patient and family that staff will carefully observe the patient for side effects and develop strategies for managing unpleasant side effects such as dizziness or restlessness. Nursing interventions to increase adherence can occur in groups or with individuals and may include motivational interviewing, cognitive techniques, and the use of standardized scales to increase the patient's insight into the benefit of medication (Sousa 2008). Nursing research has found that rehospitalization is significantly lowered for patients who participate in three or more compliance therapy sessions while hospitalized (Tay 2007).

When a patient appears to comply with oral administration of medication yet no improvement in the patient's mental status occurs, nursing staff should be alert to the possibility that the patient is not ingesting the medication. In this case, mouth checks with every administration of medication should be performed, although they are no guarantee that the medication has been ingested. Elixir preparations or rapidly dissolving tablets should be prescribed if possible for any patient who has a history of refusing medication. In anticipation of discharge, the treatment team should be cognizant that minimizing the number, cost, and daily dosage of medications enhances medication adherence. Long-acting, injectable forms of antipsychotic medication may be the preferred route of administration for patients who have residual cognitive impairments or multiple hospitalizations precipitated by medication nonadherence. Support and prompts from family are beneficial in maintaining the patient's medication regimen after discharge. Pill boxes, calendars, and regular phone or e-mail check-ins with nursing staff are all strategies used to enhance treatment adherence after the patient has left the hospital.

Nursing Care for Patients Undergoing ECT

Pre-ECT

The nursing care of the patient who will undergo ECT follows the same principles as preparing a patient for day surgery (see Table 9–6).

Table 9–6. Nursing care for patients undergoing electroconvulsive therapy (ECT)

Confirm that consent form is signed, dated, and placed in medical record
Ask patient if he or she understands the risks and benefits of ECT
Confirm that no liquids or food were taken after midnight or 6 hours prior to ECT
Remove dentures, metal in head area, and contact lenses
During procedure, monitor vital signs and cardiac function, and suction patient as needed
After ECT, remove bite block, position patient on left side, and continue to monitor vital signs and cardiac function
When patient is conscious, assess memory and inquire regarding nausea, headache, or other physical discomforts

Nursing staff confirm that a written consent form has been signed, dated, and placed in the medical record. Prior to ECT, nursing staff ask the patient if he or she understands the risks and benefits of ECT. If the patient is hesitant about the treatment or verbally indicates a wish not to proceed with treatment, nursing staff immediately notify the psychiatrist and ECT treatment team. Any patient who indicates to the nursing staff ambivalence about the treatment, even after providing written informed consent, should not be prepped by the nursing staff for the procedure. If the patient undergoes ECT as an outpatient, nursing staff make sure that arrangements have been made for the patient to be accompanied home after the procedure.

ECT is generally administered in the morning if the patient is hospitalized. Nursing staff will prohibit any liquids or food after midnight or 6 hours prior to the procedure if it is ordered later in the day. The patient should be encouraged to void prior to administration of any pre-ECT medication. Cardiac medications are administered by mouth with small sips of water. All other medications ordered for morning administration will be withheld until after the ECT procedure. Any dentures, metal in the head area (earrings, necklaces, hair clips), glasses, and contact lens will be removed.

The anesthesiologist will order an anticholinergic agent to be administered intravenously or intramuscularly to decrease the potential for aspiration or bradyarrhythmias. If a patient is anxious, intramuscular lorazepam may be ordered. A bite block will be inserted in the patient's mouth to prevent biting the tongue. During the procedure, nurses will monitor the patient's vital signs and cardiac function. Oxygen will be administered under positive pressure (100%) using a mask and an oximeter to measure oxygen saturation. Nurses will suction the patient if necessary. The anesthesiologist will administer a short-acting anesthetic medication and muscle relaxant medication. The muscle relaxant causes the sensation of paralysis and prevents muscle contractions after the administration of the electrical stimulus. Nurses should ensure that the intravenous muscle relaxant is administered after the patient is completely unconscious.

Post-ECT

After the ECT treatment, nurses should remove the bite block, position the patient on the left side to minimize aspiration, and continue to monitor vital signs and cardiac function and suction the patient as necessary. Oxygen will be continued until the patient can maintain 90% saturation (Varcarolis 2006). As the patient regains consciousness, nursing staff should assess the patient's memory and inquire about nausea, headache, or other physical discomforts (Gomez 2008). Nurses should check the patient's gag reflex prior to administering any medications or fluids by mouth. If the patient begins to exhibit signs of postictal delirium and becomes agitated, intravenous benzodiazepine may be administered (with a doctor's orders) (Gomez 2008).

In general, the preparation, monitoring, and post-ECT evaluation of the patient take approximately 1 hour. Many patients are fatigued after the procedure and should be allowed to rest or nap. All patients should be encouraged to recover in a quiet, subdued area on the unit or in their home. Following ECT, patients will experience short-term memory loss or confusion for recent events. All patients will require the nursing staff or family members to gently reorient them. Short-term memory loss generally resolves in 2 weeks but may continue for up to 2 months (Gomez 2008).

Special Considerations for Postpartum Patients With Psychotic Depression

Women with postpartum psychotic depression may have thoughts of harming their baby or other children and/or themselves (see Chapter 10, "Special Populations and Issues"). Nurses should be careful to assess women with postpartum psychotic depression for the presence of suicidal and homicidal ideation. Feelings of hopelessness, shame, and guilt are common among women with postpartum depression (Cutcliffe and Barker 2002). Partners of women with postpartum depression also can feel overwhelmed with the responsibility of parenting while their partners are hospitalized (Meighan et al. 1999). Nursing staff can provide the patient and her partner with realistic expectations about caring for a newborn, knowledge about the biological basis of postpartum depression and psychosis, and meaningful feedback about progress the mother is making toward recovery (Beck 2006). Visits with the newborn provide additional opportunities for psychiatric nurses to encourage and coach the new mother in her efforts to parent her baby.

Breast-feeding is considered the preferred method of nutrition for newborns. The mother's levels of prolactin and oxytocin are markedly increased with infant suckling, and breast-feeding may protect women from depressive symptoms (Spatz and Pugh 2007). Although the health benefits to the infant are particularly well documented, the skin-to-skin contact during breast-feeding also promotes bonding and nurturing between the infant and the mother (Spatz and Pugh 2007).

Postpartum women who are taking psychotropic medication may be hesitant to breast-feed because of concerns about the possible impact of these medications on the child's health and brain development. No psychotropic medications have been approved by the U.S. Food and Drug Administration for use by mothers who are lactating (Menon 2008). Monoamine oxidase inhibitors, clozapine, lithium, gabapentin, buspirone, zaleplon, and eszopiclone are contraindicated for mothers who are breast-feeding (Menon 2008).

The American Academy of Pediatrics (2001) released a policy statement warning that it is not possible to predict the long-term effects of antidepressants, even when taken in low concentrations, on the neurodevelopment of breast-fed infants. The American College of Obstetricians and Gynecologists recommends that all selective serotonin reuptake inhibitors or selective norepinephrine-serotonin reuptake inhibitors be avoided if possible during pregnancy (ACOG Committee Opinion 2006). In general, when the mother is taking any psychotropic medication, nurses and the mother should closely observe the baby after breast-feeding for any changes in the infant's responsiveness or gastrointestinal distress (Beck 2006).

Infants' liver, renal, and cardiac function should be checked prior to breast-feeding and periodically during breast-feeding (Menon 2008). If a mother is taking selective serotonin reuptake inhibitors, nurses should also be alert to any signs of pulmonary hypertension in the infant (Chambers et al. 2006). Mothers who want to minimize their infants' exposure to medication can pump their breasts immediately before taking their medication and feed the baby with the expressed breast milk. The nurses' duty is to provide the mother with the latest evidence-based information on the impact of psychotropic medications on breast-fed infants and to ensure that she has thorough knowledge of the risks and benefits of treatment.

Case Management

Patients recovering from psychotic depression often require a case manager to coordinate services and ensure that patients continue to follow the treatment regimen after discharge. Psychiatric home care services improve the patient's compliance with treatment and functional ability and decrease hospitalizations and demand for urgent care (Nielsen 2000). If the patient is in a residential or long-term-care facility, case managers can confer with the staff to make sure that the patient's condition is stable or consult with the nursing staff about recommendations for behavioral management if the patient experiences changes in mental status. Participation in day programs, self-help groups, sheltered workshops, and partial hospital programs helps to minimize social isolation for the patient living independently and provides additional support for the family. Case managers can also access respite services for family or loved ones who feel burdened by the responsibility of caring for the patient recovering from psychotic depression.

The goal of the case manager is to promote the patient's wellness and recovery by coordinating psychiatric and rehabilitation services in the community. Case managers confer with the psychiatrist about the patient's needs for housing, rehabilitation and vocational services, and health insurance coverage and eligibility, and coordinate follow-up care with other medical or nursing specialists. Notably, the factor most associated with effective case management is regular communication and timely information sharing between the psychiatrist and the case manager (Simpson 2007).

Key Clinical Points

- Nursing risk assessment requires the nurse to develop a therapeutic alliance and to assess the patient for suicidal ideation and potential for violence.

- For risk assessment, the nurse should obtain collateral information from the patient's family and friends and from referral sources.
- Nurses should address patients' medical illnesses and somatic complaints.
- Management of patients' comorbidities and somatic complaints requires nurses to monitor vital signs and fluid intake and output.
- In assessment of medication efficacy and side effects, the nurse needs to identify target symptoms.
- The nurse should be mindful that patients with psychotic depression often keep their delusional thinking to themselves.
- The patient should be monitored for potential drug–drug interactions.

References

ACOG Committee Opinion No. 354: Treatment with selective serotonin reuptake inhibitors during pregnancy. Obstet Gynecol 108:1601–1603, 2006

American Academy of Pediatrics, Committee on Drugs: The transfer of drugs and other chemicals into human milk. Pediatrics 108:776–789, 2001

Beck CT: Postpartum depression. Am J Nurs 106:40–50, 2006

Buchanan-Barker P, Barker P: Observation: the original sin of mental health nursing? J Psychiatr Ment Health Nurs 12:541–549, 2005

Chambers CD, Hernandez-Diaz S, Van Marter LJ, et al: Selective serotonin-reuptake inhibitors and risk of persistent pulmonary hypertension of the newborn. N Engl J Med 354:579–587, 2006

Cutcliffe JR, Barker P: Considering the care of the suicidal client and the case for "engagement and inspiring hope" or "observations." J Psychiatr Ment Health Nurs 9:611–621, 2002

Gomez GE: Electroconvulsive therapy: present and future. Issues Ment Health Nurs 25:473–486, 2008

Guy W: ECDEU Assessment Manual for Psychopharmacology, Revised (DHEW Publ No ADM 76-338). Washington, DC, U.S. Department of Health, Education, and Welfare, 1976

Koehn CV, Cutcliffe JR: Hope and interpersonal psychiatric/mental health nursing: a systematic review of the literature, part I. J Psychiatr Ment Health Nurs 14:134–140, 2007

Meighan M, Davis MW, Thomas SP, et al: Living with postpartum depression: the father's experience. MCN Am J Matern Child Nurs 24:202–208, 1999

Menon SJ: Psychotropic medication during pregnancy and lactation. Arch Gynecol Obstet 277:1–13, 2008

Nielsen M: Case management in psychiatric disability. Case Manager 11:80–83, 2000

Schröder A, Ahlström G, Larsson BW: Patients' perceptions of the concept of the quality of care in the psychiatric setting: a phenomenographic study. J Clin Nurs 15:93–102, 2006

Shattell MM, McAllister S, Hogan B, et al: She took the time to make sure she understood: mental health patients' experiences of being understood. Arch Psychiatr Nurs 20:234–241, 2006

Simpson A: The impact of team processes on psychiatric case management. J Adv Nurs 60:409–418, 2007

Sousa S: The LORS-Enabled Dialogue: improving insight in psychotic illnesses. J Psychosoc Nurs Ment Health Serv 46:44–51, 2008

Spatz DL, Pugh LC; American Academy of Nursing Expert Panel on Breastfeeding: The integration of the use of human milk and breastfeeding in baccalaureate nursing curricula. Nurs Outlook 55:257–263, 2007

Straker D, Correll CU, Kramer-Ginsber E, et al: Cost-effective screening for the metabolic syndrome in patients treated with second-generation antipsychotic medication. Am J Psychiatry 162:1217–1221, 2005

Sullivan AM, Barron DT, Bezmen J, et al: The safe treatment of the suicidal patient in an adult inpatient setting: a proactive preventive approach. Psychiatr Q 76:67–83, 2005

Sun FK, Long A, Boore J, et al: A theory for the nursing care of patients at risk of suicide. J Adv Nurs 53:680–690, 2006

Tay SE: Compliance therapy: an intervention to improve inpatients' attitudes toward treatment. J Psychosoc Nurs Ment Health Serv 45:29–37, 2007

Varcarolis EM: Manual of Psychiatric Nursing Care Plans: Diagnoses, Clinical Tools and Psychopharmacology. New York, Saunders/Elsevier, 2006

Recommended Reading

Beck CT: Postpartum depression. Am J Nurs 106:40–50, 2006

Gomez GE: Electroconvulsive therapy: present and future. Issues Ment Health Nurs 25:473–486, 2008

Koehn CV, Cutcliffe JR: Hope and interpersonal psychiatric/mental health nursing: a systematic review of the literature, part I. J Psychiatr Ment Health Nurs 14:134–140, 2007

10

Special Populations and Issues

Postpartum Psychotic Depression

Diagnosis, Recognition, and Assessment of Postpartum Psychotic Depression

During the postpartum period, women appear to have an increased risk for developing psychotic depression, and when it develops, it is often a psychiatric emergency. Periodically, one hears reports of a psychotically depressed woman who murders her children because she believed they were inhabited by the devil and had to be killed to be saved. For example, in Texas in 2001, Andrea Yates filled a bathtub with water and systematically drowned her five children. She explained during her confession that she needed to be punished because she was not a good mother and the children were "not developing correctly." Although she was initially convicted of capital murder, in July 2006, a

Houston jury of six men and six women found her not guilty of murder by reason of insanity.

Postpartum depression, or depression that occurs soon after having a baby, occurs in 13% of women who deliver (O'Hara and Swain 1996). The most serious postpartum disorder is postpartum (puerperal) psychosis, which occurs following 1 in every 500–1,000 births and is associated with mood disorders such as psychotic depression and bipolar disorder (Chaudron and Pies 2003). It requires immediate treatment. The onset is usually within a month of giving birth, but the time to presentation can be longer (Kendell et al. 1987). Risk factors include previous postpartum psychotic or nonpsychotic depression, previous major depression, psychosocial stress, inadequate social support, and previous premenstrual dysphoric disorder (see Table 10–1).

As summarized in Table 10–2, the symptoms of postpartum psychotic depression include sad mood, anxiety, initial insomnia, appetite changes, fatigue, poor concentration, agitation, feelings of maternal inadequacy, inability to enjoy the new baby, and thoughts of harming the infant. In addition, the woman often has delusions and/or hallucinations involving the baby (e.g., "The baby is inhabited by the devil" or "The baby is not mine"). The woman may also feel suicidal and may consider killing her infant and young children—not from anger, but from a desire not to abandon them. At times, the first indication that the woman is delusional may be from reports that the woman is exhibiting bizarre behavior or extreme disorganization of thought or behavior.

Because the first signs of postpartum psychotic depression may not occur until after the woman and baby are discharged from the hospital, obstetricians, pediatricians, and family members may play a key role in identifying that something is wrong that requires referral to a mental health professional. A woman experiencing psychosis can appear well temporarily, fooling health professionals and caregivers into thinking that she has recovered, but she can continue to be severely depressed and ill even after brief periods of seeming well. An accurate diagnosis of postpartum psychotic depression, like any diagnosis of psychotic de-

Table 10–1. Postpartum psychotic depression

1–2 per 1,000 births
Onset within a month of giving birth
Risk factors:
Previous postpartum psychotic or nonpsychotic depression
Previous episodes of major depression
Psychosocial stress
Inadequate social support
Previous premenstrual dysphoric disorder

pression (see Chapter 5, "Diagnosis and Assessment"), is critical so that appropriate treatment can be administered. During the postpartum period, psychotic depression is frequently mistaken for nonpsychotic depression (if the delusional thinking is missed or not prominent) or schizophrenia (if the psychotic symptoms or bizarre behavior is prominent and the depressive symptoms are missed). The former misdiagnosis can lead to treatment with antidepressants without an antipsychotic, and the latter can lead to treatment with an antipsychotic without the antidepressant. Both misdiagnoses may lead to a failure to consider electroconvulsive therapy (ECT) as a possible treatment.

As outlined in Table 10–3, the initial evaluation of a woman suspected of having postpartum psychotic depression requires a thorough history, a physical examination, and laboratory investigations to exclude an organic cause. Important tests include a complete blood count; measures of electrolytes, blood urea nitrogen, creatinine, glucose, vitamin B_{12}, folate, and calcium; thyroid function tests; urinalysis; urine culture if the patient has fever; and a urine drug screen. A careful neurological assessment is essential; this includes a computed tomography or magnetic resonance imaging scan of the head to rule out the presence of a stroke related to ischemia (vascular occlusion) or hemorrhage

Table 10–2. Signs and symptoms of postpartum psychotic depression

Sad mood	Feelings of maternal inadequacy
Anxiety	Inability to enjoy the new baby
Initial insomnia	Thoughts of harming the infant
Appetite changes	Delusions/hallucinations involving the baby
Fatigue	Bizarre behavior
Poor concentration	Extreme disorganization
Agitation	

(uncontrolled hypertension, ruptured arteriovenous malformation, or aneurysm). The stroke patient is differentiated from the patient with psychotic depression by a history of hypertension or preeclampsia, evidence of a fluid and electrolyte imbalance, and complaints of severe headache, unilateral weakness, sensory deficits, and even seizures with the neurological event (Sit et al. 2006).

Treatment of Postpartum Psychotic Depression

Frequently, a woman suffering from postpartum psychotic depression will require hospitalization because of suicidal ideation, homicidal ideation, or an inability to care for herself. The somatic treatment of an episode of psychotic depression in the postpartum period is no different from the treatment at other times of a woman's life (see Chapter 6, "Treatment"). The first decision the clinician faces when treating a patient with psychotic depression is whether the patient should be prescribed medication or ECT. The decision depends to a large extent on the clinical situation and personal preferences of the patient. The pros and cons of ECT and of an antidepressant–antipsychotic combination are outlined in Table 6–1 in Chapter 6, "Treatment." Additional considerations for patients in the postpartum period are breast-feeding

Table 10–3. Evaluation of a patient with postpartum psychotic depression

History	Folate
Physical examination	Thyroid function tests
Complete blood count	Calcium
Electrolytes	Urinalysis
Blood urea nitrogen	Urine culture (if fever present)
Creatinine	Urine drug screen
Glucose	Neurological assessment
Vitamin B_{12}	Computed tomography or magnetic resonance imaging scan of brain

and the association of postpartum psychotic depression with bipolar disorder (Chaudron and Pies 2003).

All psychotropic medications are excreted in breast milk. Thus, if the mother is breast-feeding, ECT would offer an advantage over medications for the first 2–4 weeks of the postpartum period. However, as discussed in Chapter 6, immediately after ECT is completed (i.e., in 2–4 weeks), the woman would need to begin psychotropic medication treatment. When psychotropic medications are used, the lowest effective dose of antidepressant and antipsychotic should be prescribed for the lactating mother. Observation of the infant's behavior before the mother is treated will also permit clinicians to avoid misinterpreting the infant's typical behavior as potentially related to the prescription of psychotropic medication (Wisner et al. 2002). (For excellent reviews of the use of psychotropic medications in the postpartum period, see Chaudron and Pies 2003 or Wisner et al. 2002.)

Patients and their families should be informed about the symptoms of postpartum psychotic depression, treatments, expected outcomes, and strategies to prevent recurrence. Psychoeducation will enhance the therapeutic alliance with the patient and strengthen the patient's decision-making process about treatment and her feelings of self-efficacy and mastery over her illness (Sit et al. 2006). After the patient is stabilized, a careful discharge plan should be developed before the patient leaves the hospital. Referral to intensive outpatient therapy (or a day program), along with closely spaced outpatient follow-up visits, is advisable for the first several weeks after discharge. These measures will facilitate the patient's return home and allow the clinician to closely monitor treatment response and detect clinical worsening early. Treatment plans work best when they are individualized for each patient and include interventions that have provided a good response in the past. Clinicians should encourage patients and their partners to enlist the help of family, friends, or doula services to reduce the affected mother's burden and allow her to regain sleep and recover from illness (Sit et al. 2006). Patients and their families should be advised to call the clinician if symptoms recur before their next appointment. Supportive psychotherapy that begins prior to hospital discharge may incorporate parenting skills and early infant interventions to address maternal–infant bonding and infant development (Sit et al. 2006). In-home services can also optimize outcomes for both mother and infant. Other psychotherapy options, such as family-focused therapy or cognitive-behavioral therapy (see Chapter 6, "Treatment"), are effective adjunctive treatments for postpartum psychotic depression.

Women who have had an episode of postpartum psychotic depression are usually concerned about the possibility of a recurrence if they become pregnant again. In studies of nonpsychotic postpartum depression, after one postpartum episode, the risk of recurrence of an episode of nonpsychotic depression for future pregnancies is 25% (Wisner et al. 2001). No studies have been done for psychotic depression in particular, but given the serious morbidity and mortality of an episode of psychotic depression, if a woman with a history of postpartum psychotic depression becomes pregnant again, it will be important for the woman, her family, and her treating clinicians to be alert to the possibility of its recurrence. Certainly, preventive therapy after delivery should be considered for women with a history of postpartum psychotic depression. Postpartum management should include monitoring for recurrence, with a plan for rapid intervention if indicated and/or prophylactic medication treatment.

Suicide Risk in Patients With Psychotic Depression

Studies have generally observed (although there is not uniform agreement) that rates of completed suicide and suicide attempts are higher in patients with psychotic depression than in patients with nonpsychotic depression. Patients with psychotic depression also tend to use more violent means, such as setting themselves on fire, hanging, shooting, or jumping under a train. Certainly, the symptom profile of patients with psychotic depression makes suicide a serious concern: these individuals are suffering from severe depressive symptoms and often have nihilistic-type delusions (i.e., delusions that bad things are going to happen). Unfortunately, as discussed in Chapter 5 ("Diagnosis and Assessment"), psychotic depression is frequently not recognized, and this can lead to an underappreciation of the risk of suicide. A missed diagnosis also can lead to less than optimal treatment and thus prolong the patient's recovery time, which in turn may increase the risk of suicide. In addition, many patients with psychotic depression feel paranoid and tend to internalize their thoughts, including their suicidal thoughts and ideation, making it more difficult for clinicians to assess these patients' risk for suicide.

Completed Suicide

Studies that have examined the rate of completed suicide in psychotic depression are summarized in Table 10–4. The risk for suicide in psychotic depression has been reported to be 5.3 times higher than in nonpsychotic depression (Roose et al. 1983). This finding was based on a retrospective study, covering a 25-year period, of patients who

Table 10–4. Risk of completed suicide in patients with psychotic depression

Study	Sample	Risk in psychotic vs. nonpsychotic depression
Coryell and Tsuang 1982	Inpatient sample followed for 34+ years	No difference
Roose et al. 1983	Inpatients	Psychotic depression: fivefold higher risk
Robins 1986	Psychological autopsy	15.9% of suicide victims with affective disorder had psychosis
Wolfersdorf et al. 1987	Inpatient sample followed for 0–3 years	No difference (very few suicides in either group)
Black et al. 1988	Inpatient sample followed for 2–13 years	No difference
Isometsä et al. 1994	Psychological autopsy	Psychotic depression: more likely to involve violent means (88% vs. 59%, P=0.03)

committed suicide while hospitalized on an inpatient unit. Of the 14 patients with unipolar endogenous depression who committed suicide, 10 had had psychosis. Psychosis was significantly more prevalent among the depressed suicide victims than among living depressed control subjects. The investigators concluded that the presence of psychotic symptoms was among the most powerful predictors of suicide in patients with endogenous depression. They further hypothesized that the higher rate of suicide may be an intrinsic part of the psychotic depressive syndrome.

Robins (1986), on the basis of a psychological autopsy study of 134 suicides that occurred in the 1950s, reported that 15.9% of the suicide victims with affective disorder had psychotic symptoms. The study did not separate out patients with unipolar disorder from those with bipolar disorder. In another psychological autopsy study, Isometsä and colleagues (1994) reported that patients with psychotic depression were more likely to use violent means of suicide than were patients with nonpsychotic depression (88% vs. 59%, $P=0.03$).

Three studies followed outpatients who had previously been hospitalized on inpatient units (Black et al. 1988; Coryell and Tsuang 1982; Wolfersdorf et al. 1987). In these long-term cohort studies, no difference in suicide risk was observed between patients with psychotic depression and those with nonpsychotic depression.

Suicide Attempts

Studies that have examined the rate of suicidal ideation and suicide attempts in psychotic depression are summarized in Table 10–5. The reported risk of suicide attempts varies considerably from study to study, from a 2.6-fold increase in risk (Hori et al. 1993) to no increase in risk (Lykouras et al. 2002). In a study of inpatients, Nelson and colleagues (1984) reported a greater risk of suicidal ideation in patients with psychotic depression than in patients with nonpsychotic depression. Miller and Chabrier (1987), also in a study of inpatients, found that the risk of a suicide attempt was 1.5 times higher in patients with psychotic depres-

Table 10–5. Risk of suicide attempts and suicidal ideation in patients with psychotic depression

Study	Sample	Risk in psychotic vs. nonpsychotic depression
Nelson et al. 1984	Inpatients	Psychotic depression: increased suicidal ideation
Miller and Chabrier 1987	Inpatients	Psychotic depression: risk of suicide attempts 1.5-fold higher (not statistically significant)
Johnson et al. 1991	Community sample	Psychotic depression: risk of suicide attempts greater than twofold higher
Hori et al. 1993	Inpatients	Psychotic depression: greater risk of suicide attempt and suicidal ideation; also more likely to use violent methods
Thakur et al. 1999	Inpatients/outpatients	Psychotic depression: increased suicidal ideation, intent, and attempts
Lykouras et al. 2002	Elderly inpatients	No difference
Lee et al. 2003	Inpatients	Psychotic depression: higher risk of suicide attempts

sion than in patients with nonpsychotic depression, although the difference was not statistically significant. In the Epidemiologic Catchment Area study, patients with psychotic depression had a greater number of attempted suicides and lifetime hospitalizations than did nonpsychotic depressed patients (Johnson et al. 1991). Findings from several other studies (Hori et al. 1993; Lee et al. 2003; Thakur et al. 1999) indicated that patients with psychotic depression had a greater risk for suicide attempts and/or suicidal ideation than did patients with nonpsychotic depression. A study in the geriatric population did not find a difference between patients with psychotic depression and those with nonpsychotic depression (Lykouras et al. 2002).

Two studies (Hori et al. 1993; Isometsä et al. 1994) found that patients with psychotic depression were more likely to use violent methods of suicide than were patients with nonpsychotic depression, but another study (Lykouras et al. 2002) did not find patients with psychotic depression to have an increased risk of using violent methods. This difference may be related in part to patients' age, because geriatric subjects were used in the study by Lykouras and colleagues (2002), whereas the subjects in the other two studies were considerably younger (Hori et al. 1993; Isometsä et al. 1994).

Summary of Studies of Suicide, Suicide Attempts, and Suicidal Ideation

The preponderance of the evidence base suggests that compared with patients with nonpsychotic depression, patients with psychotic depression have higher rates of suicide and suicide attempts and are more likely to have suicidal ideation. The combination in psychotic depression of a depressed mood and nihilistic or paranoid delusions makes suicide a serious concern. The fact that many patients with psychotic depression are reluctant to discuss their thoughts with a clinician until they develop a trusting relationship makes assessing the patients' risk for suicide particularly challenging.

Patients With Treatment-Refractory Psychotic Depression

The concept of treatment resistance in psychotic depression is difficult to define. Some studies have reported that as few as 17% of patients recover with treatment and remain well for 12 months (Parker et al. 1991). Furthermore, relapse or recurrence has been reported in 50%–92% of patients with psychotic depression (Aronson et al. 1987, 1988; Helms and Smith 1983; Lykouras et al. 1985; Nelson and Bowers 1978; Spiker et al. 1985). Because there is no accepted definition of treatment resistance in psychotic depression, for the purposes of this discussion, I define *treatment-refractory psychotic depression* as a psychotic depression that has not responded to an adequate trial of ECT or an antidepressant–antipsychotic combination. To determine whether a patient has treatment-resistant psychotic depression, the clinician should consider four questions (see Table 10–6).

Were the Doses of Medication Adequate?

According to recent data discussed in Chapter 6 ("Treatment"), only 5% of patients with psychotic depression receive an adequate combination of an antidepressant and an antipsychotic (Andreescu et al. 2007). These findings show a persisting low rate of adequate treatment of psychotic depression and little change from a study published a decade earlier that also reported inadequate medication treatment of patients with psychotic depression (Mulsant et al. 1997). Patients in these studies were often prescribed inadequate doses of the antidepressant, the antipsychotic, or both.

Were the Medication Trials of Sufficient Duration?

The largest studies of the medication treatment of psychotic depression were for 8 weeks (Rothschild et al. 2004) and 12 weeks (Meyers et al. 2008). Given that patients with psychotic depression may respond more slowly to antidepressant therapy than do patients with nonpsychotic de-

Table 10–6. Treatment-resistant psychotic depression

Were the doses of medication adequate?
Were the trials of medication of sufficient duration?
Has lithium augmentation of the antidepressant/antipsychotic been tried?
Was the course of electroconvulsive therapy adequate?

pression (Schatzberg and Rothschild 1992), treatment-resistant patients with psychotic depression may benefit from continuing on the medications for a longer duration, if clinically possible.

Has Lithium Augmentation of the Antidepressant–Antipsychotic Combination Been Tried?

As discussed in Chapter 6, "Treatment," in a few uncontrolled studies, lithium augmentation has been shown to increase efficacy of an antidepressant–antipsychotic combination in patients with psychotic depression. Thus, in a patient who has obtained only a partial response to the combination of an antidepressant and antipsychotic, lithium augmentation of the combination could be tried. Lithium augmentation has been studied in these combinations: desipramine and perphenazine, desipramine and haloperidol, and fluoxetine and perphenazine (see Chapter 6, "Treatment").

Was the Course of Electroconvulsive Therapy Adequate?

What constitutes an adequate trial of ECT cannot be precisely defined (see Chapter 6, "Treatment"). However, given that studies have indicated much lower ECT remission rates (i.e., 30%–47%) in patients in community settings (Prudic et al. 2004), if a patient with psychotic depression reports that he or she had an ineffective trial of ECT in the past, the clinician should obtain the medical records from the facility where the previous ECT treatments were rendered and review them to determine how many treatments were received and whether they were unilateral or bilateral. A retrial of ECT with a greater number of treatments and with more bilateral (than unilateral) treatments than the patient received previously may be indicated.

Children and Adolescents

Given the findings from the studies of psychotic depression of early onset (i.e., under the age of 25) (Akiskal et al. 1983; Strober and Carlson 1982) discussed in Chapter 5, "Diagnosis and Assessment," the presentation of psychotic depression in a child or adolescent is very likely to be an early manifestation of bipolar disorder. Like many other medical or psychiatric illnesses, psychotic depression is a poor prognostic sign when it manifests in a child or adolescent. The normal psychological development of the child or adolescent can be seriously disrupted by an episode of psychotic depression. As discussed in Chapter 5, Quinlan and colleagues (1997) found that compared with adolescents with nonpsychotic depression, adolescents with psychotic depression had a higher frequency of comorbid posttraumatic stress disorder (PTSD), and the majority of the patients with PTSD had a history of sexual abuse. Adolescent inpatients with psychotic depression also had more frequent and severe suicidal ideation than did adolescent inpatients with nonpsychotic depression (Quinlan et al. 1997).

Unfortunately, no studies have been done to guide the clinician as to the optimal treatment of psychotic depression when it occurs in a child or adolescent. Because ECT would not likely be used in a child or adolescent, the clinician is most likely to prescribe medications. However, the U.S. Food and Drug Administration (FDA) has not yet approved any medication treatments for children or adolescents with psychotic depression; only fluoxetine has an FDA indication for the treatment of nonpsychotic depression in children and adolescents. Thus, the clinician is left to extrapolate from studies of antidepressant–antipsychotic combinations in adults with psychotic depression (reviewed in Chapter 6, "Treatment").

Seniors

A considerable amount of the research on the diagnosis and treatment of psychotic depression has been done in the geriatric population. As discussed in Chapter 5 ("Diagnosis and Assessment"), the prevalence of psychotic depression may be as high as 45% in samples of elderly patients with major depression (Meyers and Greenberg 1986; Post 1962). Older patients with psychotic depression exhibit more guilt (Baldwin 1995; Lee et al. 2003); more depressive symptomatology, as measured by the Hamilton Rating Scale for Depression (Baldwin 1995; Gournellis et al. 2001; Kivela and Pahkala 1989; Lee et al. 2003); and more cognitive and functional impairment (Lee et al. 2003). Older patients with psychotic depression tend to exhibit more delusional beliefs of somatic and impending disaster content and delusional beliefs of poverty (Gournellis et al. 2008).

Many of the treatment studies of psychotic depression using either ECT or medications have either included or focused entirely on individuals with late-life psychotic depression (see Chapter 6, "Treatment"). In the National Institute of Mental Health's recently completed Study of the Pharmacotherapy of Psychotic Depression (Meyers et al. 2008), which compared olanzapine monotherapy with olanzapine–sertraline combination therapy, remission rates in young adult and geriatric samples were comparable.

Key Clinical Points

- Psychotic depression can occur during the postpartum period, and when it does, it is frequently a psychiatric emergency.
- Patients with psychotic depression have higher rates of completed suicide and suicide attempts than patients with nonpsychotic depression and tend to use more violent means.
- If patients appear to have treatment-resistant psychotic depression, clinicians should consider whether medication trials have

been of sufficient dose and duration and whether the course of electroconvulsive therapy has been adequate.

- Although many studies of the diagnosis and treatment of psychotic depression have been done in the geriatric population, few studies have been done in children and adolescents.
- Psychotic depression in a child or adolescent is likely to be an early manifestation of bipolar disorder.

References

Akiskal HS, Walker P, Puzantian VR, et al: Bipolar outcome in the course of depressive illness: phenomenological, familial, and pharmacologic predictors. J Affect Disord 5:115–128, 1983

Andreescu C, Mulsant BH, Peasley-Micklus C, et al; for the STOP-PD Study Group: Persisting low use of antipsychotics in the treatment of major depressive disorder with psychotic features. J Clin Psychiatry 68:194–200, 2007

Aronson TA, Shukla S, Hoff A: Continuation therapy after ECT for delusional depression: a naturalistic study of prophylactic treatments and relapse. Convuls Ther 3:251–259, 1987

Aronson TA, Shukla S, Hoff A, et al: Proposed delusional depression subtypes: preliminary evidence from a retrospective study of phenomenology and treatment course. J Affect Disord 14:69–74, 1988

Baldwin RC: Delusional depression in elderly patients: characteristics and relationship to age at onset. Int J Geriatr Psychiatry 10:981–985, 1995

Black DW, Winokur G, Nasrallah A: Effect of psychosis on suicide risk in 1,593 patients with unipolar and bipolar affective disorders. Am J Psychiatry 145:849–852, 1988

Chaudron LH, Pies RW: The relationship between postpartum psychosis and bipolar disorder: a review. J Clin Psychiatry 64:1284–1292, 2003

Coryell W, Tsuang MT: Primary unipolar depression and the prognostic importance of delusions. Arch Gen Psychiatry 39:1181–1184, 1982

Gournellis R, Lykouras L, Fortos A, et al: Psychotic (delusional) major depression in late life: a clinical study. Int J Geriatr Psychiatry 16:1085–1091, 2001

Gournellis R, Oulis P, Christodoulou C, et al: Delusional beliefs in psychotic depression vary according to age of onset. Int J Geriatr Psychiatry 2008 Mar 26 [Epub ahead of print]

Helms PM, Smith RE: Recurrent psychotic depression: evidence of diagnostic stability. J Affect Disord 5:51–54, 1983

Hori M, Shiraishi H, Koizumi J: Delusional depression and suicide. Jpn J Psychiatry Neurol 47:811–817, 1993

Isometsä E, Henriksson M, Aro H, et al: Suicide in psychotic major depression. J Affect Disord 31:187–191, 1994

Johnson J, Horwath E, Weissman MM: The validity of major depression with psychotic features based on a community sample. Arch Gen Psychiatry 48:1075–1081, 1991

Kendell RE, Chalmers JC, Platz C: Epidemiology of puerperal psychoses. Br J Psychiatry 150:662–673, 1987

Kivela SL, Pahkala K: Delusional depression in the elderly: a community study. Z Gerontol 22:236–241, 1989

Lee TW, Tsai SJ, Yang CH, et al: Clinical and phenomenological comparisons of delusional and non-delusional major depression in the Chinese elderly. Int J Geriatr Psychiatry 18:486–490, 2003

Lykouras E, Christodoulou GN, Malliaras D: Type and content of delusions in unipolar psychotic depression. J Affect Disord 9:249–252, 1985

Lykouras L, Gournellis R, Fortos A, et al: Psychotic (delusional) major depression in the elderly and suicidal behaviour. J Affect Disord 69:225–229, 2002

Meyers BS, Greenberg R: Late-life delusional depression. J Affect Disord 11:133–137, 1986

Meyers BS, Flint AJ, Rothschild AJ, et al; for the STOP-PD Study Group: The efficacy of combination pharmacotherapy compared to atypical antipsychotic monotherapy for major depression with psychotic features (Symposium 68C), in Syllabus and Proceedings Summary, American Psychiatric Association Annual Meeting, Washington, DC, May 3–8, 2008. Washington, DC, American Psychiatric Association, 2008, p 179

Miller F, Chabrier LA: The relation of delusional content in psychotic depression to life-threatening behavior. Suicide Life Threat Behav 17:13–17, 1987

Mulsant BH, Haskett RF, Prudic J, et al: Low use of neuroleptic drugs in the treatment of psychotic major depression. Am J Psychiatry 154:559–561, 1997

Nelson JC, Bowers MB: Delusional versus unipolar depression: description and drug response. Arch Gen Psychiatry 35:1321–1328, 1978

Nelson WH, Khan A, Orr WW: Delusional depression: phenomenology, neuroendocrine function, and tricyclic antidepressant response. J Affect Disord 6:297–306, 1984

O'Hara MW, Swain AM: Rates and risks of postpartum depression: a meta-analysis. Int Rev Psychiatry 8:37–54, 1996

Parker G, Hadzi-Pavlovic D, Hickie I, et al: Psychotic depression: a review and clinical experience. Aust N Z J Psychiatry 25:169–180, 1991

Post F: The Significance of Affective Symptoms in Old Age. New York, Oxford University Press, 1962

Prudic J, Olfson M, Marchus SC, et al: Effectiveness of electroconvulsive therapy in community settings. Biol Psychiatry 55:301–312, 2004

Quinlan PE, King CA, Hanna GL, et al: Psychotic versus nonpsychotic depression in hospitalized adolescents. Depress Anxiety 6:40–42, 1997

Robins E: Psychosis and suicide. Biol Psychiatry 2:665–672, 1986

Roose SP, Glassman AH, Walsh BT, et al: Depression, delusions, and suicide. Am J Psychiatry 140:1159–1162, 1983

Rothschild AJ, Williamson DJ, Tohen MF, et al: A double-blind, randomized study of olanzapine and olanzapine/fluoxetine combination for major depression with psychotic features. J Clin Psychopharmacol 24:365–373, 2004

Schatzberg A, Rothschild AJ: Psychotic (delusional) major depression: should it be included as a distinct syndrome in DSM-IV? Am J Psychiatry 149:733–745, 1992

Sit D, Rothschild AJ, Wisner KL: A review of postpartum psychosis. J Womens Health (Larchmt) 15:352–368, 2006

Spiker DG, Stein J, Rich CL: Delusional depression and electroconvulsive therapy: one year later. Convuls Ther 1:167–172, 1985

Strober M, Carlson G: Bipolar illness in adolescents with major depression: clinical, genetic, and psychopharmacologic predictors in a three- to four-year prospective follow-up investigation. Arch Gen Psychiatry 39:549–555, 1982

Thakur M, Hays J, Krishnan KR, et al: Clinical, demographic and social characteristics of psychotic depression. Psychiatry Res 86:99–106, 1999

Wisner KL, Perel JM, Peindl KS, et al: Prevention of recurrent postpartum depression: a randomized clinical trial. J Clin Psychiatry 62:82–86, 2001

Wisner KL, Parry BL, Piontek CM: Postpartum depression. N Engl J Med 347:194–199, 2002

Wolfersdorf M, Keller F, Steiner B, et al: Delusional depression and suicide. Acta Psychiatr Scand 76:359–363, 1987

Recommended Reading

Chaudron LH, Pies RW: The relationship between postpartum psychosis and bipolar disorder: a review. J Clin Psychiatry 64:1284–1292, 2003

Rothschild AJ: Management of psychotic treatment-resistant depression. Psychiatr Clin North Am 19:237–252, 1996

Sit D, Rothschild AJ, Wisner KL: A review of postpartum psychosis. J Womens Health (Larchmt) 15:352–368, 2006

Wisner KL, Parry BL, Piontek CM: Postpartum depression. N Engl J Med 347:194–199, 2002

Index

Page numbers printed in **boldface** *type refer to tables or figures.*